FAMILY
and
FERTILITY

FAMILY
and
FERTILITY

PROCEEDINGS OF THE FIFTH NOTRE DAME
CONFERENCE ON POPULATION, DECEMBER 1–3, 1966

Edited by WILLIAM T. LIU

With a Preface by GEORGE N. SHUSTER

UNIVERSITY OF NOTRE DAME PRESS
NOTRE DAME – LONDON

CONTENTS

PREFACE

The Conference on Population Problems which this book records is the fifth so far held at Notre Dame in the hope of throwing some light on one of the most serious of contemporary concerns. It differs from the others in two respects: first, it brought together a considerable number of distinguished scientists and social scientists who have undertaken research in this field; and, second, it was open to the public and to the press. The conference was ably planned by Professor William T. Liu, director of the Institute for the Study of Population and Social Change in the University of Notre Dame. We are also deeply indebted to him for editing the volume.

Perhaps this preface can be of some service to the reader as it offers a kind of survey of the total scope of our conferences and of the research sponsored in preparation for them. What we undertook primarily was to arrange for a confrontation between moral theologians and social scientists. It was our hope that working together they could mutually clarify their views. We tried in other words to set the challenge in a moral context, being quite mindful of the fact that since the Second Vatican Council every specifically Catholic conception of that challenge must include the whole human race, in its various groupings and its diverse commitments.

We may identify four issues. The first grows out of the

basic urges which psychologists describe at least in part—urges which alone can give moral reflection a living dimension. One of these results from the projection of oneself against the absence of oneself. Having done a small favor for a student, I received a letter of thanks indicating that in his opinion I and his Wyoming great-grandfather had been his two greatest benefactors. The comparison in terms of age doubtless seemed to him quite right. But when I questioned him about the benefactor part, he said, "You see, the only way my great-grandfather could get his girl to marry him was to march her to the altar with a gun in her back. And if he hadn't done that I wouldn't be here." The circumstance that without parental cooperation one would not have been here is a sobering thought, however naive it may be in terms of sociological statistics. Add some of the other basic urges—the desire to project oneself into the future of the race, the readiness to prove one's masculinity or femininity to the rest of the world, the almost universal affection for babies—and you have summoned up a complex of population factors which have deeper roots than ethical or demographic speculation. If you visit some parts of our country, the area around Fort Dodge, Iowa, for example, where the population is prosperously rural and traditionally religious, you will find that men and women think largely in these terms and that our urban concern with the population pressure seems to them abstract. The motivations alluded to are strong and they are universal.

The second issue is diametrically opposed to this. A few days ago I listened to a distinguished research chemist present the reasons why he had stopped working on the production of medicines to control disease and had engaged in efforts to find more effective ways to control births. In his view the postponement of death had completely destroyed the normal relationship between man and nature. No doubt he would agree with biologists like René Dubos that nature employs mysterious mechanics to control fertility. But science, he said, had now rendered these wholly obsolete. The moral problem then is basically one of trying to restore an effective balance. If the control of disease is ethically good, though it is so deep an incision into the processes of nature, then the control of population increase must be so, too. This is a conclusion reached with scientific sophistication and the available statistical evidence gives the reasoning on which it is based the quality of iron. But one may wonder if it may not be too one-sided.

The third moral issue concerns the social worker, the marriage counselor, the psychiatrist and the pastor. It may perhaps be defined quite simply as the problem of the fertile woman—the "overachiever," in Reuben Hill's phrase. Granted that St. Paul was right when he said that "It is better to marry than to burn," it would seem to follow that wedlock must provide enough sexual comradeship to put out the fire. Yet the fertile woman may produce more children than her physical and psychological endurance permit. Or she may, and this is doubtless the more important consequence, give birth to more children than she and her mate—common law or otherwise—can provide for. These are the facts and circumstances which most concern us. Various means have been employed the world round to relieve this pressure. Perhaps abortion is the one recently most relied upon. Another is the provision for relief—relief is certainly necessary—but we all know that it is not a deterrent to pregnancy. Indeed there is little we know better than we do that.

The fourth issue has to do with the intervention of the state in order to deal with the problem of imbalance—that is, the twin problems of nature versus science, and that of fertility. We may none of us feel too happy about state intervention. Bureaucracies do not always have probity and intelligence, though by and large their performance in these respects is very much better than their reputations, but they often seem to have little dogmas quite their own. Nevertheless we cannot do without them, particularly in so far as health and welfare are concerned. But private agencies do very well too; and it is essential that their abilities and efforts be correlated with what government is doing. This is only one aspect of the need for overall coordination. The problem of how best to interrelate the various agencies—say Social Security and the health services—is a very serious one, though it is less baffling than is that of bringing the poor and the illiterate into a meaningful relationship with any agency at all. These are organizational difficulties and need not concern us further here.

The moral issue involved seems to me to be this: to what extent should government agree that the scientist, as described under my second heading, be supported with public funds in order to achieve control of population increase. It is by no means a simple issue. I should like to quote from an address on "Economic Opportunities in the World of Agriculture," delivered by Professor T. W. Schultz of the University of Chicago before a United Nations Development Program Meeting on June 27, 1966. He said in part:

> Despite past economic policy mistakes and the many unresolved problems in transforming traditional agriculture, the prospects with respect to world food supplies are not as bleak as the exponential population growth curves would have us believe. These naive projections of population growth treat human beings as if they were mechanical robots when it comes to reproduction, which is patently wrong. There is underway throughout the world a fundamental change with respect to human reproduction, namely in preferences for and new possibilities of achieving effective family planning. To satisfy these preferences for smaller families much can, and should, be done in the area of modern birth control.

And he went on to add:

> The height of absurdity is revealed in a full two-page advertisement in the *Atlantic,* July, 1966 issue just out, by Olin, with its half-page heading, "Of the billion people who may starve in 1976," followed by a paragraph saying, "The statisticians say that in ten years over a billion—not a million, but a billion—people may be dying of hunger. . . ."

What this distinguished economist was saying is that the imbalance between nature and sciences is being corrected, not everywhere but pretty generally, by the introduction of methods of family limitation. We may argue about the methods employed, but virtually no one doubts any longer that the problem of population increase had to be attacked; and though many Roman Catholics might argue that rhythm is to be recommended and abortion avoided, few of them could question the fact that rhythm has played a minor part and abortion a very great one. Yet at the same time it is true that improving the food supply and effecting economic development have lagged behind. It was not necessary that this lagging should have been and still is taking place. In other words, science is not concerned with the welfare of mankind in one mode only. The energy which can now be applied to drying up the sources of hunger and disease is so great that it quite staggers the imagination.

It therefore seems evident that the moral conscience of the American citizen should be formed in the light of this duality of the scientific purpose. When it is so formed, the United States will not seem to be saying to other peoples, "the cheapest way to remove the curse of poverty from you is to have fewer of you to contend with,"—as unfortunately it occasionally does. But rather this: "An adequate food supply and sound economic progress are within reach for your children, if you have only as many as you can care for." Helping them to determine the number by offering advice and assistance is not only legitimate but actually necessary.

And so we come to the moot question as to whether "coercion" is implicit in the use of government subsidies to agencies which are helping families to cope with the problem of size. This question has nothing to do with whether penalties are to be imposed on the recalcitrant. Everybody agrees that this would be illegal and immoral. The concern is rather, is not the government in effect saying that birth control is in the national interest and that good citizenship therefore demands that you practice it? Mr. William B. Ball, general counsel to the Pennsylvania Catholic Conference, stated this position as follows, having conceded the legal right of private groups (including Planned Parenthood and Catholic rhythm clinics) to offer advice on birth control:

> It is a totally different thing to attempt to short-cut the route to such acceptance by the use of subsidies derived from the taxes contributed by all. We have particular concern over this, because we believe that if the power and prestige of government are placed behind programs aimed at providing birth

control services to the poor, coercion necessarily results and violations of human privacy become inevitable.

This objection will of course make no sense whatever to anyone who thinks that birth control is a good thing in all circumstances where Professor Hill's "overachiever" ought to do something about her problem. Mr. Ball, in his testimony before the Gruening Committee—from which this excerpt is taken—and elsewhere, takes his stance as a lawyer defending the rights of a client to privacy—in this case the urban under-privileged who, as he observes, are seldom Catholics. Never-theless it is apparent that for him, as well as for the Pennsylvania Catholic Conference which he represented, birth control is at least dubious from a moral point of view and therefore requires an explicit moral judgment of anyone who decides to practice it. That the "power and prestige of government" may therefore affect the individual's judgment is his objection.

I believe that no one seriously doubts that practicing birth control involves a moral decision. But there is a lack of agree-ment in our society as to what the judgment is based upon. A couple, having considered all the "urges" I have sum-marized under the heading of the first moral issue, may decide that having children would seriously interfere with their careers. On the other hand, a deeply religious husband and wife might conclude that since every child they have is a gift of God, any number of such gifts should be accepted, regardless of career consequences. Obviously government cannot legislate that one or both of these judgments is unten-able. All it can really say is this: some of you are well-to-do and can provide methods of birth control for yourselves if you want them, but some of you are poor and cannot pro-vide them unless they are made available to you. The gov-ernment is therefore authorizing assistance, so that you who are poor can obtain the same benefits your affluent neighbors have. Nor can the law stipulate that some methods of con-traception are illicit. It can, to be sure, refuse to sanction abortion, but this it does on quite different grounds. The government's inability so to stipulate in terms of contraception has given some Roman Catholic moral theologians a difficult time.

Nevertheless the problem has been very widely discussed, and there would seem to be a fair amount of agreement on the part of able theologians that in a pluralistic society like ours everybody has a right to that kind of birth control advice and assistance which does not violate his conscience. Planned Parenthood for its part has adopted the same position, as have other religious and ethical groups. There are any number of Roman Catholic commentaries on the question, a few of which I shall cite because they seem exceptionally well-reasoned and in some sense authoritative. The first was written for a Notre Dame conference by Father Thomas B. McDonough, of the University of Chicago, and though it deals primarily with situations existing in that city is one that admits of universal application. The second constituted the argument in favor of revising the birth control statute of Massachusetts made by Father William Kenealy, S.J., of the Boston College Law School. The third is the text of the presentation made by Father Dexter Hanley, S.J., of the Georgetown University Law School, before the Gruening Committee. The fourth is a highly cogent statement written by Father George M. Sirilla, S.J., for the *Catholic Lawyer* (Summer, 1966).

It is difficult to quote from Father McDonough's paper without doing injustice to the total logic of his position, but I shall risk it because of the pertinence of what he has to say:

> What, then, is the difference between government provision of clothing or medicine or contraceptives or cosmetics or firearms? None, whatsoever, as far as the taxpayer is concerned (for it is not his conscience that controls, but the welfare recipient's), *unless* the taxpayer can cite consequence to the public welfare that would be harmful and thus justify governmental action or refusal of action. The taxpayer can easily argue the consequences of firearms; he must also argue the consequences of contraceptives. The freedom of the individual to follow his conscience so long as he is not harming others is the paramount interest as far as governmental action is concerned. Incidentally I assume that we need not argue here that the dependent person enjoys the same freedom

and, in our society, has a claim to public assistance in order to live according to his conscience if the public assistance is reasonable and possible. In the end there is really no difference between legislation prohibiting sale of contraceptives and legislation refusing to provide contraceptives in welfare cases where the government has the task of providing, according to the conscience of the private person, what ordinarily the private person could provide. The test of proper governmental action is the same in either case: is freedom being restrained even though there is no discernible harmful effect on other citizens? In short, the government may give persons on welfare the same options that normally exist for others who are self-supporting and that are not illegal to all citizens. The factor of governmental subsidy does not change the case when government has the duty of support, as it does in the case of dependents. The principle of freedom requires that the government's substitutional support conform to the conscientious preferences of the recipients, unless those preferences are harmful to the public welfare.*

That, as I have indicated, is the tenor of the argument advanced by theologians who have expert knowledge of the law of the land. It is quite unnecessary for me to add more than one comment of my own.

The question of coercion was raised by the conference of the Bishops of the United States, meeting in Washington recently, and naturally what they said received a great deal of attention. Essentially it repeated the argument presented by Mr. Ball, though with overtones of which it seems unlikely that he would have approved. That argument is in itself quite reputable; and it is regrettable, first that it was not more effectively formulated in the Bishops' statement, and second that the statement did not take into consideration the counter-arguments so effectively advanced by Father Hanley, Father McDonough, and many others. The situation, in short, was quite different from that which prevailed at the Second Vatican Council, where the advice of the periti, the experts, was sought for and heeded.

It is wholly possible, granted human weakness, that some-

* Cf. *The Problem of Population,* vol. 2 (Notre Dame, Ind.: University of Notre Dame Press, 1964).

thing akin to "coercion" may take place in the area of birth control advice and assistance as it might in any other area of social counseling. At Notre Dame, for example, we are cooperating with the Department of Health, Education and Welfare and the Inland Steel Corporation in an effort to bring about the vocational rehabilitation of some rather aimless young men. Maybe we do "coerce" them a bit, but that is certainly better than the coercion of the reformatory. I fancy that talking a few residents of the inner city out of their patented recipes for misery, in terms of sex as well as of narcotics, might also not be too reprehensible. But finding out what is actually going on in the field of our interest might be quite salutary. It is wholly probable that the university which I represent would be willing, with some support, to work with some other reputable university, to determine as carefully as possible what coercion if any is, as a matter of fact, being exercised. In the light of the development of the social sciences, it would be a bit odd if we kept on talking about something without knowing whether it existed. Perhaps our conversation would resemble that of yore about an angel on the point of a pin.

There is no reason for being too pessimistic about the situation. The march of events is always implacable but also devious. We would despair of the future of man did we not profoundly believe that there is some good in the beast and that eventually he will be able to use that modicum of virtue for his benefit.

GEORGE N. SHUSTER

INTRODUCTION

Papers contained in this volume represent the points of view of several different disciplines about the relationships between the family system and reproductive behavior, past, present, and future. It was the aim of the Conference to bring together a number of experts in an effort to treat the common problem of sex, family, and population change; however, to achieve any kind of theoretical unity is a difficult task. Many authors who have spent a good part of their professional lives studying some aspects of family structure, human behavior, or biology were called upon to relate their work to the concerns of fertility research. Such an attempt, bold as it may be, opened up more questions than it supplied answers. A fascinating aspect of intellectual endeavors in the cultural history of man is that, as the perspectives change, new problems emerge and more meaningful and hardheaded solutions must be sought.

This Conference, like previous Notre Dame Conferences on Population, resulted in an awareness of new problems both in depth and in breadth.[1] The collective feeling seems to be that our problems overtake our answers. The need for a continuous and more rigorous dialogue among experts increases during these days as man anticipates the passing of

[1] *The Problem of Population*, I, II, III, were published by the University of Notre Dame Press in 1964 and 1965.

one era and the beginning of another. It is obvious that not only do the traditionalists and the personalists among moral theologians have difficulties in reaching an agreement as to the precise interpretation of conjugal ethics within the Catholic Church, but also empirical scientists can not readily reach a consensus as to the specific institutional or social-psychological consequences, as well as motivations, connected with the individual's choice (or the lack of it) of one method of conception control over the other.

Perhaps the broader question of change must be placed in a historical context. The *vital revolution* of population trends marks the important change between the old and the new era.[2] Not only have declining mortality rates resulted in the change of the age composition of the population, but rapid growth rates in underdeveloped countries have once more brought the Malthusian thesis into sharp focus. The pattern of a gradual population increase in early Western countries will not be duplicated in developing countries today since more effective means of disease control can be applied directly.[3] Secondly, in contrast to the laissez-faire West of the last century, governments all around the world actively intervene in various ways in trying to achieve the planned society, including the elimination of poverty and the psychological as well as physical well-being of their citizens. If the basic goal of the state is the organized, methodical advancement of the interests of its citizens, then ivy-tower social scientists must assume responsibilities in giving services to these programs in order to shape public policies in accordance with the best available scientific knowledge and with human values. On the other hand, social scientists are painfully aware of the complexities of factors surrounding the cause of a social phenomenon. Scientific findings can not always be

[2] The term "vital revolution" of population trends was first used by Ronald Freedman in his introduction to the collected essays written for the Voice of America Forum Series in 1964. Cf. *Population: The Vital Revolution* (Garden City, N. Y.: Anchor Books, 1964).

[3] Irene B. Taeuber, "The Future of Transitional Areas," in Paul K. Hatt, ed., *World Population and Future Resources* (New York: American Book Company, 1952) 25–38; Kingsley Davis, "The Unpredicted Pattern of Population Change," *Annals of the American Academy of Political and Social Sciences* 305 (May 1956) 53–59.

translated into clear-cut terms meaningful to legislators and the average layman. Conclusions derived from empirical studies, therefore, must be interpreted with great caution.

Despite the growth in research and writing on fertility and on family relations, there are a number of important gaps in the meeting of the two areas of inquiry. The considerations of family change all over the world and the unprecedented population upsurge are responsible for the new impetus to discuss the problems together. Many questions can be raised concerning the consequences of a *contraceptive society* to marriage and the family system. Does parenthood become more meaningful when the couple is free and successful in family planning? With secondary institutions taking over most child-care chores, will children become more pleasurable to parents than ever before? Will welfare and the war on poverty eventually equalize the opportunity in education and in occupational competition between middle- and lower-income families? What about the familial role structure in a *planned* and *contraceptive* society? What future changes in family functions can we anticipate when the emphasis is placed on the *conjugal* rather than on the parental role? Will new knowledge and technology in biological sciences eventually do away with the present system of family relations, as marriage, sex, and procreation become more independent of one another?[4]

Aside from these questions, there is perhaps a more immediate aspect of our concern with the relationship between sexuality and reproduction, given the prevailing human values of our society today. It is too easy to think of the change of one social fact in isolation without considering its effect on the wide spectrum of interpersonal relations, the individual's concept of self, and the hub of factors most pertinent to the acceptability of such change in this century by people of various faiths and cultural traditions.

Discoveries in human biology are more significant for the socio-psychological aspect of family life than are general economic and social development—including, perhaps, urbani-

[4] For a more elaborate discussion, see William T. Liu and Catherine Chilman, "Some Social-Psychological Considerations of Family Planning" forthcoming in the *Journal of Marriage and the Family*.

zation. Biological discoveries are more immediate in their influence on the family, and the process of diffusion does not necessarily maintain the slow pace of social and economic revolution. Application of biological discoveries, therefore, can directly change the internal environment of man; technology and economic development change the external environment, which in turn affects the values and thoughts of man.

Aside from technological innovations and the vital revolution of population growth, there is a third important force which helps to shape the family system in most societies in the world, namely: increasing government control of any type of institution which has direct bearing on family behavior. We have become more aware of the impact of such changes in the outlooks of men in various countries. Technology gives a man a sense of confidence in his capability to control his environment; it tends to change the occupational structure by making some jobs obsolete and creating the demand for others. Thus technology alters the opportunity structure, which in turn alters child-rearing patterns and educational practices after a time lag. To adapt his life to technological demands, a man must be able to anticipate the changing effect of technology and thereby plan his future. The change from "fate" to "control" orientation indeed has revolutionized the outlook of mankind.

It would be correct to assume that the desire to control the size of the family stems from the desire to improve the general lot of members already present. But to explain the actual and resultant decrease of family size by using the same reason would be an oversimplification. Men everywhere at all times desire to improve their lot, yet the actual performance varies greatly over time. Hence the desire for improvement is merely a psychological constant; the actual performance is a sociological variable. A constant can not explain a variable. In order to explain the varying degrees of commitment to limit the size of the family and the disparity of under- and over-achievement in reaching the desired number of children, one must search for answers which lie in some other variables.

One such variable—or cluster of variables—suggested by Reuben Hill in his paper is the micro-detailed structure of the family. Hill's main thesis is that: (1) family sociologists approach the problem by looking for motivational factors of individual couples in the context of role processes and decision making of the conjugal pair, and (2) by treating the family as a small social unit the investigator is able to see decision making in family planning as both an individual and a group process. The corollary of the second point is that family decisions with respect to the size of the family are analogous to family decisions on other matters.

The point raised by Hill opens a new frontier of fertility research by employing both the small-group techniques and the theory and tools of symbolic interactionists. In getting at the socio-psychological antecedents of failures and successes in family planning, the investigator must also familiarize himself with the structural aspect of the family in terms of the authority pattern, power, and affectivity between the conjugal pair, the intergenerational relations—particularly the authority of the grandmother in some cultures—and so forth. For example, in the complex of decisions which affect family size, the decision regarding the age of marriage for the young couple may involve both sets of parents. Next to be determined is how much time shall elapse between marriage and the first pregnancy. However, the parents of the couple may not have the same influence in this as in the couple's decision to marry. For each successive pregnancy and childbirth, the role of the couple's parents will also change. Hence, family size is determined by a series stochastic probability model, containing a number of irreversible decisions of, in many cases, essentially the same sets of family members.

In addition to research needed in the dynamics of family decision-making processes, there is every reason to probe into the value structure which underlies the ideal norm and provides the blueprint for the actual reality of sexual behavior. This is the topic of the papers by John L. Thomas and Harold T. Christensen. On the fundamental level, Thomas stresses the importance of sex as a basic dimension of human existence, because "of its association both with man's desire for personal fulfillment and happiness and his consequent need to establish satisfactory relationships with others. . . ." Since personal desires and fulfillment are variables which investigators must confront directly in research, to view "sex" as an isolated biological drive would only give a partial view of a very complicated problem.

To treat sex as a normative concept alone, therefore, is equally unsatisfactory when fertility behavior is examined. Psychological processes are important factors in cultural integration.[5] Thomas further stresses the fact that normative standards of sex behavior can become nebulous at a time of rapid social change. On this point, the Conference pertinently asked Harold T. Christensen to reiterate some of the questions raised in his study of normative sexual morality in three cultures: the American Mormon, Midwestern American, and Danish. The contributions made by Thomas and Christensen provide a framework for theologians and moralists in which to address to themselves some more fundamental questions with respect to: (1) the relationship between the natural law concept and the religious ideal of sexual morality, (2) the sources of the cultural ideal norm of sexual behavior in any particular society or subsociety, (3) factors determining the actual reality of sexual behavior in any society or subsociety, (4) circumstances under which the religious, the cultural, and the actual behavioral norms are equal or nearly equal, as well as conditions under which there will be the greatest gap between any two of these norms, and finally (5) cultural universals in sexual behavior and the range of restrictiveness in all known human societies. Answers to these questions may clarify related questions recurring in recent literature with respect to legitimacy, particularly in lower-income subcultures.[6]

Many of the discussions on sex, sexual behavior, and fertility patterns have their temporal dimensions. Thomas' paper attempts to trace the historical continuity of certain ideas and moral concepts. Christensen's paper focuses on the comparative nature of sexual behavior in a given time period. In order to anticipate the future, one must also assess the nature of parenthood, not just in the present but in a society which

---

[5] Cf. Francis L. K. Hsu, *Psychological Anthropology: Approach to Culture and Personality* (Homewood, Ill.: Dorsey Press, 1961).

[6] Cf. Hyman Rodman, "Illegitimacy in the Caribbean Social Structure: A Reconsideration," *American Sociological Review* 31 (October 1966) 673–83.

will be totally different from the present. What if absolute poverty is eliminated fifty, a hundred years, or two or more centuries from now? Will we argue about normative size based on present knowledge of the human family? Probably not. What if child care and other chores can be conveniently transferred to other institutions; will the change also alter the present argument for or against the normative size of the family? What if the state assumes more responsibility in educating every citizen born within its political confines; will this alter the concept of a normative size? What if all contagious diseases are controlled through better medical technology; will preventive medicine determine the normative size of the family?

Obviously none of these questions can be answered in a socio-psychological vacuum as the list of "what if's" continues. There seem to be certain laws regarding the psychic support which, in varying degree, every individual is conditioned to have. The entire mentality of family planning, perhaps, will not be a matter of "how many" is many. Rather, the question may be when to have a child and what will each additional child mean to the parents. The need would have to be individualized and the norm would have to be *privatized,* since it will be possible for the parents to control the size, the specific genetic combination, the sex, and other factors of their offspring. We probably have not given these "wild" ideas enough thought. At this Conference, however, we asked Joseph B. Tamney to look at this topic from the viewpoint of a social psychologist. Tamney's paper serves as a primary stimulus by pulling together our current thinking about the interaction between the individual and his primary relations and about the meaning of experiential existence through which we define our need to interact with others.

The gap between an overall conceptual analysis of human sexuality and the family system, and specific family behavior related to the number of children is bridged by the next three papers. In his paper Marvin B. Sussman calls for information about the differential impact of the extended kinship network in contrast to the nuclear family system on the fertility behavior of the couple. The problem is highly complicated and is difficult for the average layman to grasp because the precise functions of the extended kinship network differ from one society to another. Functions of the urban extended kinship network will have to be redefined by the demands of urban existence, which in turn may alter the family structure and relationships of its members.[7]

In carrying out a research operation, the common method of grouping family systems into the extended and the nuclear types seems to be empirically impractical or theoretically weak when one attempts to link such types to fertility behavior. First of all, during the course of socio-economic change, the process of final evolvement may not be completed at the precise point at which observations are made, and thus they may be misleading. For example, many nuclear units are physically isolated from one another yet economically interdependent, particularly at certain stages of the family cycle. Gore's study of the Indian family system in the Delhi area shows how extended kin networks are related to the nuclear unit at different times of the family cycle.[8] In the United States, parental aid to adult children in urban communities probably occurs more frequently when the young family is at the beginning stage of the cycle.[9] As the parents become older and pass the peak of their earning power, the tendency is for the adult children to contribute financially to the support of the parents.[10] Secondly, the description of a social group, such as the family type, on the basis of a slice of its content does not always give the investigator the sense of its changing characteristics and its dynamic potential. Quantitative changes in family behavior—such as in fertility patterns, age of marriage,

---

[7] Two previous papers by Sussman have elaborated the functions of kin networks in urban settings: Cf. "Parental Aid to Married Children: Implications for Family Functioning" (with Lee G. Burchinal) *Marriage and Family Living* 24 (November 1962) 320–32; "Relationships of Adult Children with Their Parents in the United States," in Ethel Shanas and Gordon F. Streib, *Social Structure and the Family* (Englewood Cliffs, N.J.: Prentice-Hall, 1965) 62–95.

[8] Madhav S. Gore, "The Impact of Industrialization and Urbanization on the Aggarwal Family in Delhi Area," (unpublished Ph.D. dissertation, Columbia University, 1961).

[9] Cf. Marvin Sussman, "Relationships of Adult Children with Their Parents in the United States," in Ethel Shanas and Gordon F. Streib, *Social Structure and the Family* (Englewood Cliffs, N.J.: Prentice-Hall, 1965) 62–95.

[10] Margaret Blenkner, "Social Work and Family Relationships in Later Life with Some Thoughts on Filial Maturity," in Shanas and Streib, *op. cit.*, 46–59.

and cohort spacing—come only long after qualitative changes have taken place within the family.

Perhaps one way to get at the relationships between the structural aspect of the family types and the differential size factor is to look at the paired relationships within the extended family system; for example, the conjugal role primacy versus the parental role primacy. In most cultures of the world today, the tendency is toward egalitarian and affective orientations between the conjugal couple with resultant changes occurring in the parent-child relationship.

Paired relations within the family may be viewed from two perspectives. The first pertains to the formally defined obligations and claims between two persons determined by age and sex status. The traditional Chinese kinship network may be used here for the purpose of illustration. In the Chinese culture, the oldest male child usually takes responsibilities early. Such responsibilities may include the education and the support of the younger siblings. The priority of financial responsibilities of the older male child may in turn determine his obligation pattern as a father. Though we do not have information about the size differential between the oldest male child's own family of procreation and those of his siblings, it is plausible that the obligation pattern may affect the number of children of each of the nuclear units within the larger extended system. Ronald Freedman gave preliminary evidence in his study of family size in Taiwan suggesting that the requisites of extended family solidarity have an effect on the number of children of each couple.[11] More rigorous research is needed to establish the precise relationship between filial obligations and the actual size of the young adult child's own family.

The second perspective for viewing paired relations within the family is on the level of an informal, nonsystem approach. Relationships between the couple, in this case, transcend the norm of the social system, yet they serve as the "screen" between the normative order and actual conjugal behavior. Sussman cogently points out that, because of the unequal

---

[11] Ronald Freedman, "Norms for Family Size in Underdeveloped Areas," *Proceedings of the Royal Society,* B. 159 (1963) 220–45.

reciprocity so characteristic of family interactional patterns, husbands and wives often consciously or unconsciously employ sex-linked personal skills to handle conflicts and consequences of such conflicts. For example, there is evidence that frequently a pregnancy occurs just prior to a couple's initial move to obtain a divorce. At any rate, sex has always been used for purposes other than the expression of love or even sensual pleasure. It can express hostility, hatred, dominance, submission, or gratitude.[12] The visceral nature of sexual reciprocity, therefore, can not always be analyzed on the normative level, for it often transcends the social system.

In the sixth paper, Fred L. Strodtbeck and Paul G. Creelan raise an intriguing question concerning family size and sex-role identity. The authors begin the paper by asking themselves: "What are the conditions under which it may be said that family size has an effect on a given characteristic?" Then, they go further and ask: "What is the nature of the family in order for the effect attributable to size to have arisen?" From preliminary evidence and data collected from several other studies by Strodtbeck and his associates, the authors suggest that the size of the family may be a built-in regulator in the process of the child's socialization in terms of sex-role identity. In the family of more than two children, as in the one-child family, the male child is provided a poor setting for the development of clear sex-role identity. While these findings are not definitive, new questions are raised concerning the psychological consequences of family size differentials.

One of the most recurring questions concerning the number of children and the *stress* atmosphere in the home has been taken up by Leon S. Robertson, John Kosa, and their colleagues at the Harvard Medical School. Following recent theories of stress etiology of illness, the authors of the paper carefully examine morbidity data collected among lower-income Bostonian families.[13] Statistical evidence suggests that family size is related to the number of morbid episodes among

---

12 The oft-quoted Chinese expression "pillow court" indicates that husband-wife conflicts as a rule are settled in the bedroom.
13 Cf. Leon Robertson and Louis E. Dotson, *Toward a Theory of Social Psychology of Illness* (forthcoming); David Dodge and Walter T. Martin, *A Sociological Theory of Illness* (forthcoming). The author is indebted to Robert-

Protestant families but not among Catholic families. The authors conjecture that this phenomenon may be explained by the fact that Catholics generally have a more favorable attitude toward large families and, therefore, do not usually perceive problems associated with the number of children as being stressful.

Definitive research is needed in many other micro-details involved in sexual interaction, family behavior, and fertility patterns.

The relationships between technology, biological discoveries, and fertility behavior also need careful attention. The traditional "natural" method of child-spacing was possible because of scientific knowledge of the ovulation cycle in women. Two questions in recent years have opened up new areas of debate. First, are there other natural means which may be more effective, more convenient, and equally acceptable? This question is well put since the rhythm method was itself the result of scientific achievement; it is conceivable, therefore, that science can offer better solutions to the problem of conception control in the future. The second question is more basic: What are the primary ends of marriage and of parenthood?

While it was not the main goal of this Conference to undertake a polemic discussion on theological questions, it was the design to include in the Conference a major section on the "actual" conceptive behavior among Catholic women in the United States and on the patterns of fertility change. Two distinguished demographers, Charles Westoff and Norman Ryder, take on both areas by supplying information which came out of their recent collaborative works. The theological stand on "acceptable" means of conception control is subject to a great deal of discussion and dispute. The social norm of family planning has been well established. Actual behavior among Catholic women, therefore, would be an acid test of the comparative strength of the social versus traditional

son and to Dodge for making the unpublished manuscripts available. Other works on this point include David Mechanic, "Response Factors in Illness: The Study of Illness Behavior," *Social Psychiatry* 1 (1966) 11–20; "The Sociology of Medicine: Viewpoints and Perspectives," *Journal of Health and Human Behavior* 7 (Winter 1966) 237–48.

demands in the area where no clear-cut, final theological word has been given. The Catholic woman now seems to be facing a more acute problem and a greater challenge to define her own course of action. The "pill," being the latest proven method, has neither been given approval nor specifically identified as "unnatural," and has probably affected Catholic couples in no lesser degree than it has affected non-Catholic couples in the United States. The evidence provided by Westoff and Ryder is convincing. The decline of fertility rates in the last few years is clear.

Voices demanding a more effective contraceptive are loudest in countries where there is greater freedom for women in obtaining employment outside the home, more egalitarianism in family relations, where decisions on family planning are more rationally based, and persons are generally more confident of man's ability to control and to alter his future. It is also in such societies that new methods of conception prevention give the population a new concept of choice—the choice of a more efficient and more convenient means in contrast to the choice formerly offered, that between a male or female-controlled means. It is conceivable that future technology in conception control will be based more on efficiency and convenience and will place under the control of the couple a larger share of the whole of human reproductive behavior and even biological processes of reproduction. A glimpse into the future is given in the paper by Anna Southam and the discussion by Gordon Perkin and Thomas Carney. Besides changes in sexual mores and attitudes and recent advances toward convenient, foolproof, and cheap means of contraception, there is a third new factor, greater knowledge of the female sexual capacity. The combination of these factors will certainly change the pattern of sexual behavior in the future. The reader may have many new questions; so do we.

What about population increase in other parts of the world today? Whether such increase will lead to a disastrous famine and human misery or whether intensified programs for reducing fertility can solve the problem is a question not directly addressed by the Conference. However, the rate of population increase, if not changed, will soon be reaching the point of serious consequences. Most authorities agree that even if there is an effective method to increase the food production in underdeveloped countries, notwithstanding political problems and social inefficiencies, the population will outdistance the food supply. This point must be driven home in a conference of this nature, for the urgency of the situation may tend to be forgotten in esoteric discussion.

Birth control programs in the Far East and in Latin America have not, in general, produced an appreciable decline in population growth. Ronald Freedman and Julian Samora present a not-so-optimistic picture of family planning. Perhaps on the whole such action failures may be attributed to an unrealistic expectation of the effectiveness of the new technology. Organizations aimed at mass fertility reduction are new social institutions. Knowledge of extremely diverse human customs, belief systems, and other influentials which affect reproductive behavior in various cultures is still lacking. It is obvious that the enormous task can not be accomplished by public health physicians and demographers alone.

Effective evaluations of existing programs also seem necessary. At the present we need to know what programs are available, where, and with what results; what factors are responsible for success in one country and failure in another; what are some of the related problems in administration, record-keeping, training of field workers, communication, and definitions of vital-statistical events; what are some of the related vital phenomena, such as abortion, miscarriage, infant mortality, illegitimacy, stillbirth, age of marriage, infecundity, and the like. A statistical summary and "progress report," ably given by Lyle Saunders, served as a concluding paper for the Conference.

As the primary organizer of this Fifth Notre Dame Conference on Population and editor of this volume, I owe a deep debt of gratitude to many individuals involved in this cooperative venture. A conference of this kind is expensive both in terms of human energy and in terms of resources needed to plan, communicate, transport the participants, and to put the results together for a wider audience. George N. Shuster, who spearheaded the Notre Dame series, deserves the credit of a major accomplishment not only in this Conference but in a number of previous conferences. Among those who have made very significant contributions to this Conference are Rev. Walter Imbiorski of the Cana Conference of the Archdiocese of Chicago, which, together with the Center for the Study of Man in Contemporary Society at Notre Dame, co-sponsored the project; Rev. Albert Schlitzer, C.S.C., of the Theology Department at Notre Dame; John Noonan of the Notre Dame Law School, and Rev. Andrew Greeley of the National Opinion Research Center. Also to William V. D'Antonio, Chairman of the Notre Dame Department of Sociology, and Julian Samora, past Chairman, the editor wishes to express his gratitude. Mrs. Gail Kowalski, Miss Sheryl Miller, Miss Ann Rice have helped in the organization and planning of this venture. And finally, without the support of the Ford Foundation these activities would not have been possible.

WILLIAM T. LIU

PART ONE

The Conceptual Framework

REUBEN HILL

1. THE SIGNIFICANCE OF THE FAMILY IN POPULATION RESEARCH

To place our subject in perspective, two extremes can be distinguished: the competing professional orientations and contributions of traditional demography as against family sociology. Demography, along with economics, has been considered one of the dismal sciences. Because the demographer was dealing with the questions of fate—such as marriage, birth, illness, and death—over which men traditionally have exercised little control, the traditional demographer has conceptualized man as a passive recipient—a particle—in the grip of physical, biological, and social forces. He has, accordingly, dealt with the phenomenon of reproduction in a fatalistic way, preferring to look at national trends, demographic rates, and the influence, over long periods, of changes in the economy and in the polity—in all of which the individual's behavior did not have to be accounted for. His units were large aggregates arrived at by joining together data by gross categories of the population. There were no living actors in his units.

The family sociologist has proceeded quite differently. He has taken as his unit of study the individual or the small

3

group and has observed its behavior under different social conditions. His observations have been at the microscopic level of individual and small group actions and decisions on issues over which man does exercise some control. He sees man as initiator as well as reactor and as capable of making decisions within the context of his interpersonal relationships in the social structure.

With man's expanding control over his environment, his demographic fate—to use a term coined by the American sociologist, Kurt Back—has also begun to come under his control. The orientation and focus of the family sociologist has, accordingly, become increasingly relevant for understanding voluntary childbearing. Indeed, the man-over-nature orientation of the family sociologist gives him an advantage over the demographer whose nature-over-man fatalism has inhibited his participation in the research required for identifying the factors to be manipulated in action programs.

Each has made his contributions to population policies and programs. The demographer has contributed at the national level by the generalizations and predictions he has made about reproductive changes and their social and economic correlates. He has further undertaken cross-national studies of large magnitude to test theories about "the demographic transition" as countries have urbanized and industrialized. He has been influential in creating, staffing, and improving national systems of statistics in most of the countries of the world, treating not only vital events but all types of information useful for predicting changes in these events. The demographer's documentation of the increasing population growth in developing countries and its implications for educational and welfare goals has precipitated the formulation of explicit policies to regulate population growth. His findings have also been used in Europe to rationalize pronatalist programs of graduated family allowances to equalize the cost of child rearing and reward couples taking on the responsibility for large families. Thus, although his findings have been descriptive and nonprescriptive, they have nevertheless lent themselves to application, because they have dealt with the same aggregates utilized by policy makers and planners at the levels of national and international planning.

In contrast, the family sociologist brings the phenomenon of population growth down to the level of the decisions or nondecisions about family size. The nation's problem with population growth rate is, thereby, decomposed into the behaviors of millions of couples coping with the timing of marriage and the number of children desired. There are families which underachieve, having fewer children than they desire; families which overachieve, having more children than they desire; families which are lucky or effective in having neither more nor fewer than they desire. The family sociologist seeks to explain this relative success or failure in family size control.

When first asked by the University of Puerto Rico to undertake a study of Puerto Rico's population problem a number of years ago, the writer was intrigued by the task primarily as a means of studying family problem solving. Puerto Rico's problem appeared not so much as a population bomb exploding in the Caribbean, although that can be documented easily enough, but as hundreds of thousands of individual families failing in the first primal task of marriage, the control of family size in line with family goals.

Puerto Rico has been a good place to observe this type of family problem solving or nonsolving because its people are extremely conscious of optimum family size, uniformly preferring two or three children, yet bearing, on the average, six—a people with small-family-size goals and large-family achievements.

The problem of overachievement, moreover, was concentrated in the lower classes of the island. Our task was to discover the factors accounting for the success of some and the failure of most lower-class Puerto Ricans to contain their fertility in line with their stated goals for family size. Later, in an educational experiment, the problem took a more active form. How could those who were unsuccessful be rendered more effective in fertility planning.

The numerous studies which had been undertaken in Puerto Rico acted as a deterrent against seeking any simple solution. A family sociologist, the present writer, was to bring his own conceptual tools to bear on the problem, which had already been examined by economists, demographers, and anthropologists. One unique contribution, at the time the

5

research was undertaken, was a view of the problem from the perspective of family heads. What did the problem of numbers look like from inside families? Our team took the position that planning the future size of the family was a function of the family itself. Government and private agency programs may suggest, advise, and facilitate, but the decision to start planning, what to do about it, and whether to continue with these actions is made by the married couple itself.

Analysis of the behavior of family units might show, therefore, why some family planning programs succeed and some fail, and how the steps in family planning are accomplished.

Finally, the challenge of this study of success in family planning was that much of what the family sociologists learned here could be used in other areas of family life. The concern of the research team was not yet primarily with the solution of the population problem in Puerto Rico and in other parts of the world. The major goal and motivation was to understand how families coped with problems. And here was one that was constantly in front of them, on the agenda all of the time. Conditions leading to effective planning of family size, it was thought, might be analogous to those which enable families to plan effectively in any field.

Let us review some of the steps that were taken to assure a family-centered study: the choice of the unit of study, the choice of an appropriate theoretical framework for formulating guiding questions and setting the limits on observations, and the construction of a schema of analytic categories encompassing the territory to be studied.

The units of observation and analysis for demographers in the general area of human fertility and its control have varied greatly—counties, states, provinces, countries, whole societies, sometimes broken down for purposes of studying differential fertility in groups stratified by income, occupation, education, and residence. Medically oriented researchers have usually focused on mothers, treating the woman as the biological unit of study, which, in turn, fits well with their conception of the problem as a special instance of maternal health.

The monumental Indianapolis study, concerned with the social and psychological factors affecting fertility, appears to have focused on wives, although they were obviously treated as reporting agents for their families. This particular group interviewed husbands, but they rarely joined these data from husbands with those obtained from wives to construct family behavior items.

At the time of the Puerto Rico study, no research team had, as yet, taken as possible units of study either reference groups or nuclear family groups. At the time of these explorations four criteria were proposed for the selection of a study and observational unit in fertility control. Working from the assumption that fertility planning was group rather than individual planning, the unit emerged as the entity of planning, choice making, and action. The unit should be capable of serving as the referent in some conceptual system or a theory if our findings were to become part of the creative theory. And the unit must be accessible for empirical observation and investigation. The unit of study should also ideally be the unit of medical and educational services in matters of fertility control.

Of the possible units considered—the individual, the marriage pair, the nuclear family group, reference groups, communities—one met all of the criteria satisfactorily, as one would expect with a family sociologist as director, the nuclear family of procreation.

Having chosen the nuclear family as a unit of study and observation, it was incumbent upon us to choose, among the many approaches to the study of the family, the conceptual framework which would most fruitfully utilize the nuclear family as a planning and decision-making association.

Seven such approaches had been developed, each with its own distinctive definition of the family, its favorite concepts, and its own body of theory. The choice seemed to lie between the structure-functional and the symbolic interaction approaches, both of which had much to contribute to the research problem. The interactional frame of reference for studying small groups seemed most appropriate, since it lends itself especially well to analysis of the family as a planning and decision-making association. Its key concepts consist of a kit of mental tools which are uncommonly useful in the study of the dynamics of human fertility. Some of these

7

concepts are status and interstatus relations which become the basis for authority patterns and initiative taking. The key concept of role is common to both the structure function and the interactional approach, and there are many modifications—role taking, role playing, role organization, role conceptions, process concepts, communication, consultation, conflict, compromise, and consensus. The interactional approach has been broad enough to capture and order the central processes involved in group planning and problem solving which need to be observed in a study of fertility dynamics. This is a large order, since they include among others, the processes of goal setting, choice among means, allocation of accountability and responsibility for actions taken, as well as built-in processes of evaluation of the successes and failures of the plan which need to be fed back as problems for a group solution and reorganization.

Finally, the interactional approach provided more than tools for observation, it provided a body of theory which can be drawn upon in the formulation of diagnostic study questions. From family interactional theory come propositions which may be used as guideposts in the quest for the social-psychological antecedents of success in family planning and control. These antecedents are different in quality from the psychological and social-economic correlates of fertility of most social demographers from the days of Indianapolis down to the present time. They pertain to the dynamic quality of interaction systems and are oriented to intergroup processes, rather than to traits, characteristics, and status categories.

Certain foci are suggested by the family interactional framework. Using it as a microscope, it is apparent that the family, if permitted, is concerned intermittently with what Robert Reed has called negative and positive control of procreation. Decisions are reached and actions agreed upon. Failures are discussed and action is taken to correct them. The process remains at the agenda level of discussion for the effective period of childbearing unless cut short by the sterilization of one, and even this would be a consequence of husband-wife interaction.

With this perception of the family as the decision-making

unit of society with respect to control of the family size, the family interaction theory suggests that the family's effectiveness as a planning unit would be a function, in large part, of the efficiency of its communication system. Thus, a likely study focus suggested by the interactional conceptual framework would be the processes of communication, the factors thought to be related to communication, conditions favoring communication, and impediments to communication which thwart goal setting, discussion, consensus, and decision making. These would receive major attention. Perhaps this is enough to illustrate the large advantage in taking a family-centered view of the issues of fertility control.

Certain aspects of the family and fertility studies in Puerto Rico and Jamaica appear to have particular relevance to family planning in other countries, notably, as illustrated in Figure 1, the schema of antecedents of fertility control.

The schema is designed to show direction of relations from left to right: the most distant on the extreme left and the closest on the extreme right. What have been hypothesized as the independent, intervening, and dependent variables in the studies of the family factors in fertility control? The social setting factors (Block A) are residence, education, occupation, type of marital union, religious affiliation, and income; these are related to effective family planning, shown as Block G, by means of five intervening sets of variables, each represented by a block in the model.

The variables shown under Block B, quite a distance away from the dependent variable, Effective Family Planning, capture what might be termed the general orientation toward change. Does the individual value change, or are the traditional ways best? Does the individual value planning, or does he believe fate determines his lot in life? Does he have high aspirations for himself and his children? Does he actually strive to achieve these aspirations? In sum, this block indicates the extent to which the respondents desired to manipulate change and to which they are actually doing so.

A third crucial block of variables (Block D) is qualitatively closely related to Block B, since it reflects values and motivations to act, but is much more specific with respect to fertility control: namely, attitudes toward family size and its control;

9

these are, therefore, placed close to Block G, Effective Family Planning. What does the individual perceive as many or few children? Does he desire many or few, or does it make little difference? If he wants few, is this desire the consequence of having many children or is it independent of such experience? When and under what conditions did he first develop a preference about family size? What are his attitudes toward limiting family size, toward methods of birth control, toward the clinics and their family planning service?

A fourth cluster, known as Block C, Information and Knowledge, involves the crucial cognitive dimension and refers to the availability of technical means for goal achievement in family size. How much does the individual know about birth control methods? What is the timing of learning about these methods? Does he know the location of the nearest dispensary, depot, or clinic? If he's either ignorant of certain methods or, as in Block D, considers them objectionable or finds the clinic unacceptable, birth control as a means of family limitation is unavailable in our sense of the term.

A fifth block, E, refers to general family organization, to the typical patterns of allocating power, responsibilities, tasks, and affection within the family. Where is the locus of power in making decisions? What is the division of tasks and responsibilities? Are the roles of husband and wife integrated or are they segregated in carrying out these responsibilities? Lee Rainwater, in a recent study, had made this the core of a typology of families: role integration and role segregation. What is the sociometric network of affectional relations, coalitions, and emotional alignment within the family? How familistic-restrictive is the family structure with respect to the wife's mobility and freedom to participate outside the home? This is what is meant by general family organization. If it is found to be related to effective fertility planning, it might also be related to other types of family planning.

Finally, consider Block F, the action potentials of the family, both with respect to coping with general problems and with respect specifically to action on family size. Is the structure of the family conducive to the implementation of joint and/or individual goals? Is there consensus on most issues

FIGURE 1 Schema Specifying the Hypothetical Interrelationships of Selected Antecedent, Intervening, and Consequent Variables in Fertility

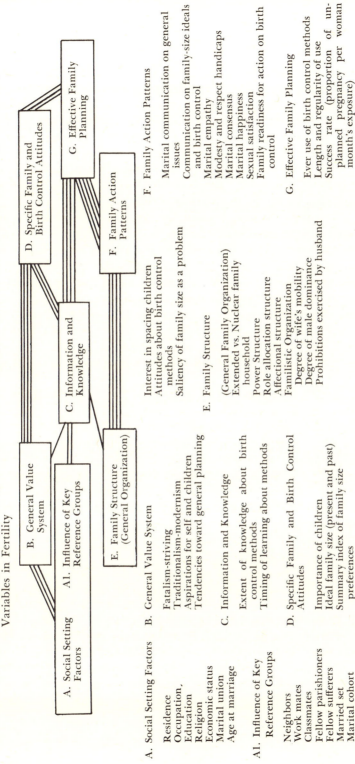

A. Social Setting Factors

Residence
Occupation,
Education
Religion
Economic status
Marital union
Age at marriage

A1. Influence of Key Reference Groups

Neighbors
Work mates
Classmates
Fellow parishioners
Fellow sufferers
Married set
Marital cohort

B. General Value System

Fatalism-striving
Traditionalism-modernism
Aspirations for self and children
Tendencies toward general planning

C. Information and Knowledge

Extent of knowledge about birth control methods
Timing of learning about methods

D. Specific Family and Birth Control Attitudes

Importance of children
Ideal family size (present and past)
Summary index of family size preferences

E. Family Structure
(General Family Organization)

Extended vs. Nuclear family household
Power Structure
Role allocation structure
Affectional structure
Familistic Organization
Degree of wife's mobility
Degree of male dominance
Prohibitions exercised by husband

F. Family Action Patterns

Marital communication on general issues
Communication on family-size ideals and birth control
Marital empathy
Modesty and respect handicaps
Marital consensus
Marital happiness
Sexual satisfaction
Family readiness for action on birth control

G. Effective Family Planning

Ever use of birth control methods
Length and regularity of use
Success rate (proportion of un-planned pregnancy per woman month's exposure)

in the family? Is this consensus realized? Are there barriers to communication on marital issues and on birth control? Is there agreement on initiative taking with respect to the crucial areas of family life, including sex relations and the timing of birth control use? It is within this Block F that the micro social-psychological factors are concentrated, the degree of husband-wife communication, the ability to arrive at consensus, the phenomenon of empathy, and the general inclination toward taking action. These are among the most important variables constituting the family's action potential. A number of studies have been undertaken utilizing the major elements of this schema originated in Puerto Rico to provide guidance for data collection and analysis.

The bibliography of readings accompanying this paper identifies some of these studies. The work in Puerto Rico, Jamaica, and Haiti, and in Belgium, France, and Greece are immediate consumers and verifiers of this schema. Lee Rainwater's work on working-class families has adopted depth interview methods similar to those used in his recent book *Family Design*. The detailed findings cannot be presented here, but a factor analytic condensation of findings is given in Figure 2, based on the Puerto Rican survey phase. It is significant that communication has emerged as the "hub variable." Several of the variables which had a high zero relationship to fertility planning effectiveness show up in the factor analysis primarily by virtue of their association with communication. Thus, for example, factors of sexual and general marital adjustment, which have lost their direct association to fertility control through the factor analysis, retain their strong association with communication. The complex of planning-striving and fatalism shows a similar but weaker pattern. Ideas and concerns about family size also operate in a secondary fashion by their association with communication and the timing of perception of family size as a problem.

At this point, the presentation requires a less condensed treatment of the findings, concentrating primarily on the Puerto Rico and Jamaica data—the microscopic conditions associated with types of fertility planners. How do those who are family planners differ from those who are nonplanners?

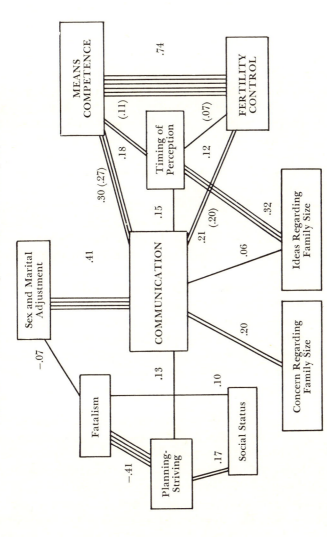

FIGURE 2 A Factor Analytic Model of Fertility Dynamics

Code: (1) Figures in parentheses are partial correlations, holding all other factors constant. All other figures are zero-order correlation coefficients.

(2) The size of the correlation coefficient is approximated by the number of lines between factors; correlations less than 0.10 are not statistically significant at the 5 per cent level.

How do those who are effective planners differ from those who are accident prone?

It is possible to distinguish those families who have at least tried out one or more birth control methods from those who have not, using the terms "ever users" and "never users." With respect to the values dimension, the more couples believe in planning their life in general, the less traditional their views, the more seriously they value small families, the earlier in their marriages they feel concern about the problem, the more likely they are to have used birth control methods. Similarly, the more egalitarian the family organization, the more communication there has been between husband and wife, the more they know each other's family size desires, the more likely they are to have tried contraceptives. In short, any values which are favorable to trying family size control and any type of family organization which makes it easier to explore solutions to problems lead to the practice of birth control.

What are the differences between casual users of birth control who are short-term, irregular, and long-term regular users or persistent users? The casual user is more likely to regard the people with few children as lucky and to be, nevertheless, higher in his perception of how many is a large family. The persistent user believes more in planning in general —uses planning in his everyday affairs more frequently and is more likely to persevere in an enterprise which he has started. But more important than these beliefs, the long-range persistent user has a family geared to more protracted cooperation. Family planning is not an individual enterprise but a cooperative one. In long-range user families, there is more discussion between husband and wife, and it is less likely that the husband's mood prevails one-sidedly in decision making.

The people most likely to use birth control regularly are, thus, primarily those who can organize effectively in general. The principal factors are emphasis on planning, communication between spouses, and ability to come to a joint decision. They tend to be a well-organized family team. The casual user couple is as much or even more aware of the pressures of a growing family on resources and tries birth control methods, but it lacks the organization to follow through and pursue the goal to a successful conclusion.

Now, three distinct syndromes of family planning are identified: the "never user" whose value system, tardiness in perceiving the problem of family size, and kind of family organization are inimical to family planning; the casual user who has some motivation for controlling family size but no capacity for sustained effort, and the long-term persistent user whose ideals about planning, concern about family size, and effective family organization make him an effective user of birth control methods.

Still a fourth type of family planner has favorable attitudes toward birth control and a modern outlook but lacks the family organization to achieve the protracted cooperation so necessary to the successful use of birth control. These are families who have been sterilized—about one-sixth of Puerto Rican families. On the traditionalism-modernism continuum, the sterilized are on the modern end. The wife is permitted to work outside the home. They feel it is better to struggle against odds than to resign oneself to fate and that a child should make his own place in the world rather than follow in his father's footsteps. They believe in planning, but they actually tend to let nature take its course as far as day to day planning goes. They are, on the average, as well informed on birth control as are long-term users of birth control. It is in family organization that the sterilized appear more similar to the never users. Communication between spouses is lower; the husband tends to be dominant in most affairs, especially in reaching a decision after a disagreement. The husband is more likely to misperceive his wife's interests and ideas, and, vice versa, the wife is more likely to misunderstand and misinterpret her husband than are long-term persistent users of nonsurgical methods.

The sterilized are, thus, among the most modern in general values and most tradition-bound in family organization. Hence, if they feel the pressure of many children, it is not surprising that they use a method which does not entail any future cooperation, although it is still drastic and unconventional. This type of family reflects a set of attitudes widespread in Puerto Rico and in many other parts of the world,

15

and it probably explains the popularity of sterilization—a one-time method—as the method of birth control.

In brief summary, we have shown that the following are important for effective planning of family size: (1) a generally modern value system, (2) definite views favoring small families, (3) sufficient information about birth control, and (4) an efficient, flexible family organization.

For successful fertility planning, the efficiency of the family must be tuned to a strong motivation. If the motivation is weak and the type of family organization is rigid or ineffective, providing a barrier to planning, planning will not occur. Here values and family organization are in negative relation to the goal. With increase in the strength of motivation arising with higher parity women, ineffectual attempts at birth control would be made. If the motivation is very strong while the family structure impedes planning, effective measures which require no planning—like sterilization or, in some countries, abortion—may result. There values are positive, but family organization is negative. In the developing countries, all three of these properties—motivation, information, and effective family organization—are lacking in couples, particularly early in their marital careers. Ideals about family size are often not crystallized until later in the marriage. Knowledge of methods, for example, was not acquired until after the third child in Puerto Rico and Jamaica. Communication on most matters having to do with the issue of family size did not occur until late in the marriage. Couples need to share their values and their knowledge about family size control early in the marriage, but even in the United States there is a tendency to start family planning late and casually until the number desired is reached, using contraception to close a family or sterilization, as in Puerto Rico, or, as in many developing countries of Latin America, abortion. Fortunately, these features of family organization can be sufficiently changed by education and persuasion to bring about an increase in the proportion of effective planners, as we have shown in two field experiments in Puerto Rico and Jamaica.

The direct attack on the question of family organization which concentrates on widespread premarital education for marriage and parenthood, improving the competence of men and women in communication, in group problem solving, and in understanding the opposite sex, should be considered as much an integral part of a fertility planning program as the disseminating of contraceptive information and the elimination of prejudice about the use of birth control methods. Moreover, the by-product of happier families might be valuable in its own right.

With this overview of the important contributions which family structure and dynamics make in determining the success of fertility planning, let us look at the chief global irreversible decisions affecting the reproductive career and the actors involved in these decisions. The writer acknowledges the stimulation of Charles Westoff in this concept of the irreversible decision. What irreversible decisions are made over the reproductive career which affect fertility directly and who are the chief decision makers? First, there is the decision about when to marry. In closed marriage systems the parents make the decision; in open systems, the couple make it with parents participating. The second decision is how soon to have the first child. Here the couple, parents, and peers are often involved. The phenomenon of pregnancy before marriage and its consequences are detailed by Freedman and Coombs.[1] This question, how soon to have the first child, has tremendous consequences in economic achievements, ultimate family size, and family stability. Whether to use birth control methods to effect intervals between births is still a third irreversible decision: couple, parents, pastor, and medical personnel may all enter into the act. A fourth issue, what methods to use, will involve the couple, pastor, and medical personnel. When to have the second child: couple, parents, peers. How many children to have: couple, parents, peers. And, therefore, when to close a family: couple, parents, sometimes medical personnel.

Present family planning programs the world over deal with very few of these decisions. There is no work on the timing of the decision to marry, virtually no work on the timing of

---

[1] Ronald Freedman and Lolagene Coombs, "Childspacing and Family Economic Position," *American Sociological Review* 31 (October 1966) 631–48.

the first birth, very little on spacing intervals for subsequent births. The focus of action programs has been upon closing the family and upon what methods to use. Reaching women of high parity primarily late in the marriage is, as someone has said, "closing the window after the bird has flown." The argument is made that motivation is highest for high-parity women and there will be diffusion from such women to women of lower parity. This is entirely plausible but has not yet been convincingly demonstrated.

What about the decision makers reached in the worldwide family planning campaigns? In clinical programs where maternal health is the rationale in family planning, the decision maker reached is the wife, as if the decision were the wife's alone. And this is true in patriarchical societies as well as in societies where women are more likely to be free agents. The husband is rarely seen, as though he had no stake in the matter, whereas we know that he is the most influential referent in Puerto Rico, for example. Donald Bogue shows him to be equally influential in his Chicago studies. Moreover, in Western countries the methods most used in the past have been male methods, *coitus interruptus* and the condom, rather than female methods. This ought to be indication enough as to where the motivation is in family planning. No family planning programs have yet been aimed at couples as such, yet they are the chief decision-making unit with respect to sexual relations and birth control use. Posters all over the world invite not couples but mothers to the clinics with the admonition: "Mothers, for your children's sake and for your health, come to the clinic." Even when the poster shows the father standing by the mother, he is seen as a passive image. Parents of couples appear very rarely to be taken into account. An exception, here, is the wise-grand-mother poster shown in Taiwan. The grandmother in the poster is looking across at her son and his small family of two children, saying, "Don't you wish that *your* children would be so wise," or words to that effect. It is unique. And yet, in almost all of these countries, grandmothers are especially important in decisions on when to marry and when to have the first child.

In our Puerto Rican studies, the second most important

referent, after the husband, is the wife's mother. She was both the most important one and the first to suggest that maybe the couple had had enough children. Moreover, if you ask husband or wife from whom they would like to hide the fact that they are using birth control methods, they reply that it is the mother. So she serves both as the conscience, the inhibitor, and the second most important instigator in taking action.

Peer groups are just beginning to be reached, as in Chicago and Alabama where Bogue's organization of neighborhood "coffee sips" is oriented to the age peers of the couple. In India the depot holders of contraceptives indicate the peers that they feel they can influence, and they are building up their clientele through those they can influence.

Medical personnel and pastors as influentials have been largely ignored in family planning campaigns except in training programs for clinicians. The surveys show that physicians in private practice are both uninformed and obstructionists in some countries. In Morocco, there seems to be a division of labor in which the public health physicians put in the IUD's and the private physicians take them out. In that particular program the private physicians were not even invited to the National Seminar on Family Planning. The medical corps will either work for you or against you. They cannot be treated as neutral or indifferent.

In Catholic countries the clergy have been viewed as hostile to family planning, but few attempts have been made to win their cooperation, despite abundant evidence from the initiatives taken by many influential Catholic groups that this would be a profitable alliance to establish. In the Moslem countries of Turkey, Egypt, Tunisia, and Morocco the leading imams have been given authoritative statements from the theologians asserting the compatibility of family planning with the teachings of the Koran. As a consequence, there has been little evidence of obstruction from religious sources. But in general, our programs of education and mass-communication as well as our direct contact—door to door programs—have ignored all decision makers except the "little woman." And in some countries she is the most cloistered member of the family. Now, it must be recognized that working at several decision levels with a diffuse audience of decision makers would attenuate one's messages, if carried out all at once. But experimental programs which dealt with the newly marrieds and their parents might be compared fruit-fully with the somewhat stereotyped high-priority programs now monopolizing our resources.

In quick summary, what has been covered? Opening with an orientation to the contrasting stances of the demographer and the family sociologist, we indicated the contributions the latter brings to the population problem: namely, the identifi-cation of the micro-familial properties necessary before any contraceptive technology developed will be adopted and effectively used. We took account of some of the problems faced by the family sociologist in seeking to make a contribu-tion to the body of knowledge needed for more effective fer-tility control. We provided a rationale for making the family the unit of study and action, and outlined the advantages of symbolic interaction as the conceptual framework for view-ing the problem. We continued with a list of the micro-fam-ilial properties required, as involving high motivation, mast-ery of the means, and an effective family organization for taking action on family goals, all three of which appear to be lacking in familes of the developing countries and in couples everywhere early in their marital careers. A schema was devel-oped which clustered these properties into six blocks of var-iables which constitute the crucial explanatory variables accounting for differential fertility control effectiveness.

The findings from the Puerto Rican data, treating factors analytically, were reviewed revealing adequacy of husband-wife communication as a central explanatory factor, when all other factors were held constant, in determining success in fertility planning. From the same studies, we distinguished different types of users of contraceptive methods—the "never user," the "quitter" or "casual user," the "regular long-term user" and the sterilized—showing the propensity for general planning and acceptance of small-family-size norms, accom-panied by communicativeness in spouses and egalitarian rela-tionships. I characterized ever users as against never users, but also distinguished between casual users and long-term users. The sterilized were shown to have strong motivation, but ineffective family organization, forcing them late in the marriage to undertake a method which didn't require cooperation. A field experiment, based upon these findings, has demonstrated the feasibility of changing family ineffectiveness by education to improve fertility planning, arguing for the equal importance of such programs with information and persuasion programs designed to effect levels of knowledge and motivation.

Closing with the identification of seven irreversible fertility-related decisions and the chief decision makers involved in these decisions, we argued for making a beginning at organizing more ambitious programs of action which would increase both the number of the decision levels and number of crucial decision makers reached in social action programs.

SELECTED READINGS

Back, Kurt W., Hill, Reuben, and Stycos, J. Mayone. "The Puerto Rican Experiment in Population Control." *Human Relations* 10 (November 1957) 315–34.

———. "The Dynamics of Family Planning." *Marriage and Family Living* 18, no. 3 (August 1956) 196–200.

Berelson, Bernard, *et al. Family Planning and Population Programs.* Chicago: University of Chicago Press, 1966.

Blake, Judith. "Family Instability and Reproductive Behavior in Jamacia." In *Current Research in Human Fertility.* New York: Milbank Memorial Fund, 1955. Pp. 24–41.

Carisse, Colette. *Planification des Naissances en Milieu Canadien-Francais.* Montreal: Les Presses de l'Universite de Montreal, 1964.

Davis, Kingsley and Blake, Judith. "Social Structure and Fertility: An Analytic Framework." *Economic Development and Cultural Change* 4, no. 3 (April 1956) 211–35.

Girard, Alain and Henry, Louis. "Les Attitudes et la Conjoncture Demographique: Natalite, Structure Familiale et Limites de la Vie Active." *Population* 11, no. 1 (January–March 1956) 106–41.

Hill, Reuben, Stycos, J. Mayone, and Back, Kurt W. *The Family and Population Control.* Chapel Hill: University of North Carolina Press, 1959.

————. "Family Action Potentials and Fertility Planning in Puerto Rico." In *Current Research in Human Fertility*. New York: Milbank Memorial Fund, 1955. Pp. 42–62.

————. "La Estructura de la Familia y la Fertilidad en Puerto Rico." *Revista de Ciencias Sociales* 1, no. 1 (March 1957) 37–66.

Rainwater, Lee. *Family Design*. Chicago: Aldine, 1964.

Stanton, Howard. "Puerto Rico's Changing Families." *Transactions of the Third World Congress of Sociology*, vol. 4. London: International Sociological Association, 1956.

Stycos, J. Mayone. *Family and Fertility in Puerto Rico: A Study of the Lower Income Group*. New York: Columbia University Press, 1955.

Stycos, J. Mayone and Back, Kurt W. *The Control of Human Fertility in Jamaica*. Ithaca: Cornell University Press, 1964.

Stycos, J. Mayone, Back, Kurt W., and Hill, Reuben. "Interpersonal Influence in Family Planning in Puerto Rico." *Transactions of the Third World Congress of Sociology*, vol. 8. London: International Sociological Association, 1956.

PART TWO

The Macroanalysis of the Family and Fertility

JOHN L. THOMAS, S.J.

2. SEX, MARRIAGE, AND THE FAMILY: A REAPPRAISAL

The title of this paper inspired the rather playful thought that if I were writing at the turn of the century during the high tide of straight-line evolutionary theorizing, I would probably have been tempted to interpret the terms "sex, marriage, and the family" as marking necessary stages in the historical development of human sexuality. Proceeding on this assumption I might have made out a plausible case for man's social evolution from a primitive stage of sexual promiscuity, up through various types of mating relationship, to the gradual formation of the institutionalized family. Or, inversely, I might have traced the development from archaic man's all-encompassing extended family system, through its loss of function to competing institutions and the emergence of the nuclear family, down to contemporary Western society's preoccupation with the genital aspects of sex. If I happened to be in a specially creative mood, I might even have developed a cyclical theory of change by combining the two approaches and hypothesizing that the present trend would lead to promiscuity, followed in due time by a sexual backlash, which would lead, in turn, to more stable mating rela-

25

tionships and, coming full circle, to the eventual restoration of the institutionalized family.

Fortunately, this facile theorizing on the basis of a priori assumptions regarding the evolution of man's social institutions now stands discredited; though some might contend, and not without reason, that it has only been replaced in some circles by equally unscientific speculations of a quasi-mystical character. At any rate, among family sociologists at least, the increase of scientific knowledge has brought some measure of discretion. Our theory-building aspirations tend to be relatively modest. We are interested in studying the process of change within observable social systems, in identifying the relevant variables, and, hopefully, in discovering some causal relationships. In other words, our theorizing is confined well within what Robert K. Merton has euphemistically termed the "middle-range."

As the various papers discussed at this Conference suggest, changes that affect man's relationship to reproduction will have repercussions on his total conduct of life and, in this sense, logically require careful rethinking and restructuring of all his other relevant relationships. This requirement becomes all the more apparent if we recall that throughout most of the known past this concern with reproduction, considered in terms of both individual fulfillment and social continuity, has constituted one of the major wellsprings of organization and motivation in all human societies. Thus we may safely conclude that the introduction of social or cultural development that radically modify essential elements of this relationship will have far-reaching implications not only for the happiness and fulfillment of individual persons but also for the general welfare and progress of the whole society.

At previous Notre Dame Conferences on Population we noted that throughout much of the past it was generally assumed that the average couple were able to bear and rear all the children they might be privileged to have during the course of their marriage, though the long history of contraception, sterilization, abortion, and infanticide indicated that there were some individuals who for various reasons attempted with more or less frequency to frustrate or eliminate the reproductive outcome of their sexual relations. We

26

further discussed in considerable detail some of the major factors that had served to modify this traditional view in the West. Stated briefly, starting around the sixteenth century a series of developments in science, industry, medicine, and other areas, together with the introduction of radically new thought-ways in philosophy and theology, began gradually to transform many long-accepted Western attitudes and practices relating to standards of living, infant and maternal health care, social mobility, status of women, and the formal education of children. We also pointed out that because the consequent adjustments in sexual, marital, and family patterns were either ignored or blindly opposed, there was little awareness of the need to develop a more adequately comprehensive, integrated conception of human sexuality. As a result, most Western societies now include a wide variety of conflicting or contradictory sexual attitudes and practices, and modern man is finding it increasingly difficult to make sense of his sex-related activities. A serious reappraisal of sex, marriage, and the family is long overdue.

Sex is such a fundamental dimension of human existence, by reason of its association with both man's desire for personal fulfillment and happiness and his consequent need to establish satisfactory relationships with others either as partner or parent, that neither individual persons nor societies can long avoid clarifying their stance in its regard. Sex may mean different things to different individuals within a given society and may have different meanings for the same individual at various stages of the life cycle; yet, considered by itself, it is not this factor that makes human sexuality problematic. Past and present experience suggests that one of the major sources of difficulty in dealing with sex—and all known societies have had their share of difficulties—is the tendency to take a partial or topical view of it, to see it in terms of only one of its dimensions, and to value only one of its many aspects.

In particular, much of the confusion reflected in contemporary sexual attitudes and practices stems from our failure to view human sexuality and its expressions both as a connected whole and within the total context of the present human conditions. Following a segmented, topical approach

27

we attempt to evaluate the sexual activities of infants and children, premarital, marital, and extra-marital experiences, illegitimacy, and so on, without viewing them within the wider context of total personality development or taking into consideration their effects on the various other elements necessarily involved in securing the life-fulfillment of the individual and his responsible participation in society. Since my approach to sexuality is based on certain assumptions regarding the form and functioning of sex, marriage, and the family in a social system, I shall begin with a brief explanation of my conceptual framework.

Conceptual Framework

As I see it, the fundamental dimensions of our problem can be outlined as follows. Inasmuch as man is not man except in community—that is, the quality of being social is constitutive of human nature—men can realize their true stature in the proper fulfillment of the characteristic functions of their nature only in association with others. Thus men come together in various types of societies and associations to fulfill their needs; and because their needs are multiple and varied, men tend to establish a number of relatively distinct organized associations of an economic, political, social, religious, and sexual character to meet them. Thus every enduring society includes a set of more or less clearly defined beliefs and values relating to man and his needs, and through its specific institutions and implementing normative patterns of conduct seeks to define, regulate, and control the acceptable ways through which its members are to achieve these goals. Individual societies, of course, may differ widely in the clarity with which they define their basic beliefs and values, the consistency with which they integrate their various institutions, and the extent to which they establish and maintain adequately implementing patterns of conduct.

For purposes of the present discussion, therefore, we assume that there are things that must get done in any society if it is to continue as a going concern. These functional requisites constitute the generalized conditions necessary for the maintenance of a given social system, and while the specific social structures established to actualize them may differ from society to society, they must be realized in one way or another if the society is to endure. For example, if the members of a society refuse or are unable to reproduce, if they fail to provide for the training of their offspring, if they lack sufficient motivation to engage in communal endeavors, and so on, the society will eventually cease to exist.

The more obvious functional requisites of any enduring society appear to be adequate adjustment to the environment, provision for maintenance and replacement of resources, more or less systematic and stable division of labor, a set of shared communal goals and of means prescribed to attain them, and a system for controlling disruptive social behavior effectively. At the same time, because a society can survive only if it recruits new members, provision must be made for the adequate training of each generation so that youth will be prepared and motivated to fulfill the essential adult roles required for the maintenance of the community. In other words, because man is a social being, group life requires certain organizational features through which each individual must adjust and adapt his personal interests to the demands of others and of the ongoing social system. Every enduring society must provide adequate means for meeting these insistent interpersonal problems, so that the general organizational features we have mentioned are requisite to the continuation of social life, regardless of the cultural forms that may be employed to implement them.

Further, we assume that there exists a requisite functional relationship between various cultural elements, in the sense that one cultural element requires the other either as a necessary condition or as an inevitable consequence. This means that a quality manifested in one department of a culture requires certain particular qualities in other departments. For example, the maintenance of a technically advanced society requires, among other things, that the family, school, and social system not only provide for the adequate motivation and increased formal education of youth but also so structure their social relationships that their interests, energy, and time are not unduly diverted from the pursuit of this necessary preparation.

Considered from the viewpoint of the individual and his adequate motivation, this second assumption implies that if a given social system is to function successfully, its members must acquire the type of character traits and personal aspirations that make them want to act in the way they should act; that is, they must effectively desire to do what objectively it is necessary for them to do in terms of the social system. This does not imply that the individual must be totally immersed in society, but it does remind us that society is not wholly extrinsic to him. The "one and the many" is not an "either-or" relationship. Although the human person, as the possessor of definite rights, is properly regarded as the source of individual liberty; nevertheless, the social quality of his nature necessarily specifies the inherent limitations of this liberty. Indeed, the freedom of the individual includes several limiting aspects. Not only is it determined by the existential ends for the attainment of which the individual must be free, but the degree to which this attainment becomes possible is also limited by the conditions of the society in which he lives. As a social animal, man exercises his freedom within a community, that is, within a concrete, intricate web of social relationships that define, condition, and limit its expression. For all practical purposes, the individual will experience freedom only to the extent that this web of relationships makes provision for its development and exercise. As we shall point out, the family functions as the primary social instrument in promoting this essential socializing process, so that if a given family system becomes unable to accomplish this to any marked degree, it seems doubtful whether external force or social sanctioning could long secure effective cooperation of group members under democratic conditions.

We therefore assume that by controlling sexual behavior for purposes of reproduction and by providing for the basic socialization of offspring, the family appears in every human society as the only workable means for satisfying a series of essential human needs. Although we have limited knowledge of the adaptive potential of the human agent and have only started to explore the interrelationships between family systems and other social institutions, it now appears that no culturally advanced society can endure without some type of family system. Through the fulfillment of its distinctive functions—sexual, reproductive, educational, affective, economic, and so on—the family possesses a manifold utility that renders its universality inevitable. As a matter of fact, although the major functions fulfilled by the family are separable from one another and might conceivably be carried out by separate institutions, they are not separated in any known major family system.

In the light of these observations we may safely conclude that a sound family system constitutes a functional prerequisite for the maintenance of any enduring society and, further, that there exist requisite functional relationships between qualities or elements of a family system and those of other cultural subsystems; for the family is only one institution among others in a complex, ongoing society and must achieve relatively close integration with existing occupational, educational, political, religious, and other social subsystems if it is to meet the needs of its members. Hence, under conditions of change, the family system affects and is affected by other related institutions, while, within the family system itself, changes affecting the extended family circle require changes in the nuclear or conjugal unit and changes affecting one member's status and roles within the nuclear family unit call for corresponding changes in the statutes and roles of other members. Specifically, society-family, extended family-conjugal unit, husband-wife, and parent-child dichotomies are reciprocal. This is a trite observation, to be sure, yet our tendency to take a topical approach in studying social phenomena all too frequently leads us to ignore its obvious implications.

Further, we assume that to gain an adequately comprehensive view of human sexuality in a given culture requires, among other things, that we keep in careful focus the known or assumed "facts" about sex, their accepted individual and social implications, and the relative significance attributed to these "facts" and their implications by members of the society. Human sexuality proves to be such a complex phenomenon not only because it implies disjunctive though complementary personal attributes (masculinity-femininity) and consequently couple-centered fulfillment but also because one of the functions with which it is associated, the bearing and rearing of children, is closely related to group continuity and survival. The quality of being sexed has profound implications for both individual persons and society. Sex never appears as a merely physiological phenomenon. It is one element of the total personality, radically conditioned by this totality and the socially structured environment within which the individual develops and strives for fulfillment.

Thus if we consider sex from the viewpoint of the individual, it appears as a way of being and relating to the world and to others. As a way of being and relating to the world, it is reflected at all levels of the person's activity: psycho-physical, and spiritual (super-individual). Its way of being and relating to others is reflected in the sexually specific, culturally defined statuses and roles in terms of which boys and girls in a given society are trained and which later determine their relative social positions, accepted areas of action, and permitted aspirational goals as members of the adult community. Considered from the viewpoint of society, sex appears as the basis of that primary human community of life and love designed to provide for the mutual development and happiness of the couple, the orderly fulfillment of their sexually associated needs, and the adequate recruitment of new members of society through parenthood.

Finally, we may logically assume that in a rapidly changing, pluralist society like our own which does not clearly define its behavioral standards or institutional norms and leaves its cultural goals loosely integrated and somewhat nebulous, individuals must formulate their own "designs for living" by choosing rationally among the various patterns society offers them. In regard to sexual conduct such self-determination requires a clearly defined, personal conception of the meaning of mature sexual fulfillment and an internalized set of related value premises on the basis of which logically consistent choices can be made throughout the various stages of the life cycle. Young people can avoid normlessness and unthinking conformity, with consequent loss of individual freedom, only to the extent that they are made aware that mature self-determination necessarily implies the personal development and acceptance of a consistent set of value premises in terms of which they can evaluate alternative modes of conduct and select appropriate behavioral patterns. As the logical implications of our current pluralism become more manifest in the practical order, young people experience an increasing need for an integrated philosophy of life, for they are presented with a variety of segmented, inconsistent, frequently contradictory purposes and practices from which to choose. Although we seem reluctant to face the fact, it should be clear that a society's failure to provide the prerequisites of responsible choice can prove just as frustrating and destructive of personal freedom as the imposition of arbitrary restraints on its exercise.

HISTORICAL BACKGROUND

The fact that man is not endowed with a "sex instinct," in the sense that he does not inherit a predetermined desire to accomplish a specific behavioral goal in his use of sex—that is, his sexual goal-behavior is not innate or "built-in"— clearly indicates the importance of social definition and learning, and suggests that culturally diverse attitudes and practices relating to sex, marriage, and the family will reveal far from uniform patterns. As we learn from history, man's sexually associated relationships have been institutionalized in a wide variety of forms. In practice these constitute the culturally determined and accepted sets of obligatory normative relationships centering around the fulfillment of man's basic sexual functions as these are defined by a given human group. Nothing definite is known about the early sexual patterns of man prior to written history, and little will be discovered since the essential data are lost forever. Although there exists considerable information concerning the various stages of man's evolution as a biological species, such evidence pertains to his anatomical development and consequently provides no significant information regarding his corresponding social development. If we accept some current estimates, it appears that there has been no development in human brain size during roughly the last 100,000 years, and we may thus assume that the most significant aspect of man's later evolution has been his cultural development. On the other hand, we do not know to what extent or through what possible stages man's neural, hormonal, and mental systems may subsequently have evolved, though their evolution would definitely affect his sexual patterns.

In regard to family origins, some scientists have felt that a good deal could be learned about man's early family institutions by studying the family groupings of the anthropoids. Unfortunately, in addition to the fact that the separate ancestral line of the great apes—that is, the gorilla, orangutan, chimpanzee and gibbon—is thought to date back some 30 to 35 millions years, thus making them man's very distant "cousins" indeed, the social activities of only the gorilla and gibbon have been studied in their natural habitat, and their family groupings appear to be dissimilar. Others have assumed that the study of the family institutions of contemporary stone-age societies would throw some light on the family patterns of prehistoric Stone-Age man, yet we cannot validly conclude that contemporary stone-age and Paleolithic societies constitute similar stages in man's social evolution and consequently have similar family institutions.

On the other hand, if we move from conjecture to recorded history, we discover some functional similarities common to all stable family systems. Thus all systems include some form of mating relationship through which men and women are brought together for purposes of procreation; some form of marriage ceremony or social arrangement by means of which this mating relationship becomes publicly recognized and duly acknowledged by the community; some definite habitat, household or home in which this marital unit is localized; some organized provision for the satisfaction of the material and psychic needs associated with childbearing and the nurture of offspring; and, finally, some type of kinship system designating how persons sharing various relationships based on marriage or common descent are related to members of a given family unit and to each other.

Apart from these common general elements, marriage and family systems tend to differ considerably. Nevertheless, since they are determined in part by the individual and social needs they must satisfy if society is to survive, their form and functions cannot be regarded as wholly arbitrary. For example, a family system based on general promiscuity—that is, a system in which there would be chance, ephemeral mating relationships but no provision for couples to share life in common or provide for the rearing of their children—though hypothetically possible, does not appear feasible, and all past attempts to establish such patterns have failed. A family system based on group marriage, or the simultaneous marital union of two or more men with two or more women, also seems generally unworkable; and while some alleged examples of this pattern have been reported, they appear to be deducible either to such customs as wife-loaning and wife-sharing under specified conditions or to rather broad prenuptial and postnuptial sexual freedom. Judging from the evidence of history, therefore, we may conclude that only family systems based on some relatively stable form of monogamy or polygamy (polygyny or polyandry) are capable of meeting man's essential requirements in this regard. Of the known societies for which relevant data are available, strict monogamy is observed by a minority, polygyny is found to some extent among the majority—though among the numerically great civilizations only Islam is polygamous—and polyandry is fairly exceptional.

Considered in terms of sexual attitudes and practices, perhaps the most important difference between family systems is the relative significance they attribute to the individual nuclear unit and the extended family group. For example, in systems emphasizing the nuclear family unit composed of husband, wife, and unmarried offspring, mate selection is regarded as the prerogative of the individual and is to be based on mutual love; both lines of kinship enjoy equal status; and though relatives may exert considerable influence on the nuclear unit, their power is founded on affectional bonds and may not be vindicated directly as a right. On the other hand, in systems emphasizing the extended family the significant unit is a group of relatives, including several generations related either by marriage or blood and bound together by a clearly defined set of mutual obligations and rights. Family property rights may be inherited equally, or inherited by only the eldest son (stem family), or shared by a group of brothers and their male descendents (joint family). The individual conjugal family constitutes but one unit of the larger family system, the dominant members of which exercise considerable control over mate selection and assume major responsibility for protecting the interests of the total family group. Under these conditions, marriage is valued primarily as a means of strengthening the group, romantic love attachments are regarded as possible threats to the system, and concern with legitimacy leads to careful supervision of marriageable females.

Unfortunately, we have only limited knowledge concerning the historical development of most family systems. Among the great civilizations of the West the family initially appeared as a relatively autonomous, powerful social institution based on a stable conjugal bond, clearly defined parental control over offspring, and assured kinship support, particularly from paternal relatives. The father was unquestioned head of the family, though his authority was limited by kin control and custom. Unmarried women remained under the protection of their fathers until marriage, at which time they were placed under the protection and control of their husbands.

Generalizations are hazardous in this area, but among the known Western civilizations it appears that with the passage of time kinship support gradually lessened, the conjugal bond became less stable, and parental control less absolute. At this later stage, characterized by easy divorce, childlessness, and increasing disorganization, social controls designed to protect the weak and support family institutions were usually introduced by the state. Although no social law is implied, in all these civilizations the family tended to evolve from a strong, quasi-autonomous social institution, within which the statuses, roles, mutual rights and obligations of members were formally defined, toward a small conjugal unit enjoying only informal support from relatives and held together primarily by affective bonds.

Thus it appears that when societies increase in density, complexity, and technology, the accompanying division of labor and specialization leads to a clearer articulation or delimitation of various institutional structures and objectives, with the result that the nonessential functions of the extended family system are gradually taken over by other institutions and the character of even its essential functions tends to be modified. At the present time, since the nuclear family type with its limited formal kinship bonds and restricted family circle appears most consonant with the spatial and social mobility, individualism, and economic independence required by the increasing industrialization characterizing most modern societies, it seems safe to conclude that it will gradually emerge as the dominant type in all modern, economically developed countries.

Systems of Sexual Control

All known human societies have maintained some set of normative standards or codes defining the appropriate expressions of sex for their members. Considering the variety of beliefs, values, fears, and practical concerns that must have entered into the formulation of these codes, it is not surprising that cultures differ greatly in the ways they have defined their prohibitions and permissions in this regard. A review of the relevant cross-cultural data available indicates that past societies have followed two fairly well-defined, though not mutually exclusive, approaches in formulating their systems of sexual controls. The first may be called "society-centered," in the sense that it seeks to regulate only those expressions of sex that are considered harmful to the welfare of society. Because some control of sex is needed to maintain a society's marriage, reproductive, kinship, social status, and ceremonial systems, regulations are established in terms of these systems.

This approach is common to most cultures outside the Jewish and Christian spheres of influence. As we have noted, its point of departure is society rather than the person, and its regulations are formulated only in terms of those social phenomena with respect to which it is thought to be important. Thus, sexual relations are forbidden between certain classes of persons within the kinship group or clan; sexual advances are prohibited during certain ceremonials or at specified seasons or under designated circumstances. As a rule, these standards are formulated and enforced either to insure social order or secure divine protection. Outside the regulated areas, free sexual expression is permitted to the individual. In other words, sexual conduct becomes a moral concern when it violates the socially defined standards of the group.

The second approach may be called "person-centered," in the sense that it is concerned with the individual and his personal responsibility for all conscious use of his sexual faculties. Hence it seeks to develop normative standards that will cover all expressions of sex under all circumstances. In this personalist approach the use of sex is evaluated primarily in terms of the perfection of the person, and, in practice, sexual control will appear to focus on the sexual faculty itself rather than on those specific expressions of sex that the group may judge to be particularly disruptive of social order. In other words, the conscious use of sex will be regarded as morally good only to the extent that it conforms to what is believed to be the person's divinely designed nature and destiny.

The significant differences between these two approaches is that the first evaluates sexual conduct in terms of some other social phenomenon in respect to which it is important; the second, in terms of a definite view of the human person. In the first, only those uses of sex that have recognized social significance have moral relevance; in the second, every free, conscious use must be evaluated morally—that is, every thought, word, and action concerned with sex is regulated by a personally supervised code which is devised with respect to a creator, an integral personal destiny, and a social purpose. Both approaches produce a set of culturally standardized practices which range through definitely prescribed or preferred or permitted patterns of conduct to those definitely proscribed. In one way or another, both solve the perennial problem of reconciling the need for control with the need for expression; in each approach, however, the solution is founded on different value premises.

These two approaches have been presented in some detail because they throw considerable light on the current situation. As participants in the broad stream of Western culture, the American people have tended to follow the personalist approach, yet it is becoming increasingly clear that large numbers no longer accept the philosophical and theological assumptions upon which this approach was founded. On the other hand, since most of our contemporaries apparently find the restraints of a society-centered approach quite objectionable, the present American sexual trend can perhaps best be characterized as a confused, uneasy drift toward normlessness.

THE CHRISTIAN EXPERIENCE

Although we have pointed out above that the Christian approach to the formulation of a sexual code is personalist or person-centered, it may be useful to add a few observations concerning the total context within which Christians have developed their specifically religious conceptions of sex, marriage, and the family. Christians regard the family as a wholly secular, human reality, open to change and development. This reality, however, touches personal salvation intimately not only because individual Christians experience it in their lives but also because, according to Catholic doctrine, it has been incorporated by the Savior into the present economy of salvation and constitutes a formal sacrament. This means that Christians face the perennial challenge of analyzing and understanding the evolving form and functioning of this institution, for it is precisely this integral human reality and not some neat juridical abstraction that becomes in marriage a way of Christian perfection and a symbol of the mystery of the living communion between Christ and his church.

In most respects Christianity added little that was essentially new to existing family ideals when it was introduced into the Hellenic world. Early Christian apologetic writers could appeal to the high family morality of Christians as an argument for the faith only because their pagan adversaries recognized these values in theory if not in practice. All workable conceptions of the family must respect both the individual and social exigencies of man's dual sexual nature and procreative potential. Christianity's major contribution in this regard was to make more explicit or bring into sharper

39

conceptual relief the practical implications of these inherent requirements.

As a spiritual movement, therefore, Christianity did not attempt to destroy or replace existing family systems. Yet the gospel message relating to chastity, the equality of the sexes before God, the value of human life, and the sanctity and stability of the marriage bond exerted a gradual leavening influence on the attitudes and practices of all who accepted it. As the faith spread, the need to evaluate various alien family practices as well as to refute numerous heretical tendencies among the faithful forced Christian leaders to clarify their thinking and make more explicit some of the practical implications of their teaching regarding marriage and the family. The conceptions that finally merged were a synthesis of Christian, Jewish, Hellenic, and Teutonic elements which theologians and canon and civil lawyers had gradually shaped into the fairly consistent beliefs, values, principles, and practical norms that became embodied in Western family traditions.

On the other hand, Christian theologians have experienced great difficulty in developing an objective, conceptually integrated view of human sexuality. Thus, pre-Augustinian Christian teachers, possessing no conceptually refined, well-integrated system of moral theology and beset by various types of Gnostic, Manichaean and Pelagian heresy, were chiefly preoccupied with the pastoral problems of defending marriage and refuting various doctrinal extremes. St. Augustine's classic definition of the "goods" of marriage could have furnished the basis for a more positive theological approach, but his assumptions regarding sexual concupiscence and original sin prevented this. Briefly, he argued that inasmuch as sexuality in fallen man was vitiated by the most virulent form of concupiscence—*libido carnalis*—the marital act was not inherently good and could only be justified by the external good of procreation.

Proceeding on this assumption that sexual concupiscence was evil in itself or in its use, Christian thinkers for the next thousand years were primarily concerned with discovering extrinsic reasons for justifying marital relations and warning against excessive enjoyment even in their legitimate use.

Although more balanced countercurrents of opinion gradually began to develop after the sixteenth century, it must be noted that Augustine's pessimistic conception of sexual concupiscence has run like a leitmotif through most past Christian thinking on sexuality until very recent times and has consequently inhibited theologians from developing a balanced view of marital relations.

Moreover, although conjugal love has always been highly esteemed in the Christian tradition, it has only relatively recently been formally conceptualized as a value meriting special attention. Conjugal love is not a univocal term, of course, and our conceptions of it, as of all relationships between man and woman, are culturally conditioned and consequently admit of a wide variety of meanings and expressions. In one form or another and in varying degrees of intensity, conjugal love is found in all known cultures, As presently understood in our society, however, it requires *de facto* as well as *de jure* equality of partners; and since the cultural and social changes making possible the enhanced status of women are fairly recent, this may partially explain its past relative neglect in official circles. At the same time, in a nuclear-type family system conjugal love plays a strategic role in assuring the stability of marriage, so the central position theologians now assign it may reflect their awareness of contemporary conditions.

Finally, throughout most of the Christian past there has been little understanding or appreciation of feminine sexuality and little concern with the wife's enjoyment of marital relations. This is frequently explained as the result of religiously induced feminine prudery and a predominantly male-centered approach to sexuality, yet these explanations lack adequate cultural perspective. Given the absence of scientific obstetrical assistance during childbirth and the distressingly high maternal and infant mortality rates characterizing most of the past, together with the lack of any reliable and morally acceptable means of separating marital relations from conception, it should be obvious that women would develop different views of sex than men and would consequently tend to regard marital relations primarily as an inevitable burden, the prelude to suffering, sorrow, and danger. Under these

41

conditions, it is not surprising that the wife's expression of conjugal love in marital relations came to be defined as the dutiful proferring of the marriage "debt," an obligation to which moral theologians and spiritual directors devoted considerable attention.

At the same time, once knowledge and acceptance of various contraceptive birth control techniques became widespread, religious leaders reacted by placing primary emphasis on the right performance of the act as the major criterium of acceptable marital relations. Their concern with the negative aspects of the act—a typical example of that doctrinal imbalance that frequently occurs when cherished moral standards come under attack—while it did not wholly ignore the changing significance of feminine sexuality, tended to leave its positive implications largely unexplored.

A REAPPRAISAL

The aim of this somewhat lengthy though hopefully not too tedious exposition has been to prepare the ground for a critical reappraisal of human sexual phenomena. If our assumptions regarding the social nature of man are substantially correct, it seems clear that we cannot develop an adequately comprehensive conception of human sexuality without taking into consideration its social conditioning and inherent relationships to existing marriage and family institutions. Further, if man does not possess a sex instinct, his sexual goals and conduct are not biologically predetermined and consequently offer a wide scope for the exercise of creativity, freedom, and responsibility. The purpose of our brief historical review was to show the relatively wide spectrum of sex, marriage, and family patterns that different societies have devised and found more or less workable.

Moreover, if men develop their definitions of what is right or wrong in the practical order within a broader framework of value referents which are organized into fairly consistent general schemes and related to their conceptions of the nature of man and society, the sexual codes and standards that men approve will depend not only on their perceived personal and social needs but also on their underlying beliefs about the nature and purpose of life. All such codes have their "costs," considered in terms of training and the limitation of spontaneity; for in order to be effective, they must regulate sexual conduct in more or less detail throughout the life cycle and, at the same time, meet the relevant institutional demands of the total social system.

As products of the Western cultural stream, our views of sex, marriage, and the family are the result of a long historical development characterized by marked changes in the family system and consequently in the statuses and roles of family members, by extensive scientific advances in our knowledge of man's reproductive faculties and sexual behavior, and by new philosophical and theological insights regarding the inherent dignity of the human person. We are also beginning to acquire some awareness of the unique human value and significance of conjugal love; of the specially unifying, affective, relational importance of sexual relations in expressing and fostering this love; and of the crucial, yet increasingly demanding functions of parenthood under modern conditions. Because these latter developments, in particular, have proceeded more or less separately and have not been fully integrated into any of our existing sexual codes, they tend to generate needs and expectations that are not consonant with these codes and consequently lead to frustration rather than fulfillment.

This underlines the current, pressing need for a careful reformulation of existing sexual standards and codes. To be adequate, such a reformulation must be based on a thorough reinterpretation of the personal and social significance of sex, together with a consistent restructuring of the various relationships relevant to its meaningful development, expression, and regulation. In other words, we need a reformulation of human sexuality that will take into account the mutually complementary character of its psycho-physical, psycho-social and spiritual qualities, the various stages of sexual growth in the process of personality development, and the individual and institutional implications of sexual relations as a unique means of expressing human love and creativity. Obviously, the contributions of religion, philosophy, and the various medical and social sciences are required here, for no single

43

discipline can adequately deal with the complex phenomena involved. Although the development of a workable sexual code may rightly be regarded as a continuous process, it should be clear that no healthy society can long ignore this ongoing challenge and remain content merely to drift.

Before proceeding to indicate the direction that a valid reappraisal must take, it may be well to note that mere "viewing with alarm" or negative criticism serves no useful purpose. Many contemporary critics avoid facing the real issues by having recourse to a convenient type of scapegoating, in which Puritanism, Jansenism, Victorianism, or even Christianity itself become the chief villains in the piece. But scapegoating is not analysis. Shallow ranting against the assumed or real inadequacies of past beliefs, attitudes, and training does not provide the basis for a positive program of action. No religious, ethical, or social system has created sex. Human sexual phenomena are insistent "givens" which we must somehow try to make sense of and deal with accordingly. Mere rejection of past codes and standards solves no problems. The basic issues relating to the understanding and control of sex remain constant and must be confronted.

Considered in a Christian context, a valid reappraisal must begin with a clarification of the meaning of sex as we presently understand it in the light of revelation, reason, research, and experience. Hence our basic starting point should be full acceptance of the fact that the Creator made man a sexed person, "male and female he created him," and regarded his creation as good. This means that the quality of being sexed is an essential attribute of the human person—a person's essential way both of being and relating to others and to the world. Moreover, since man was created with a dual sexual nature (male and female), the quality of being sexed in the individual person can be fully understood only in relation to a reciprocal "other" sex, and it is ultimately on the basis of, or in terms of, this relationship that we define the meaning of sex in theory and practice.

Further, the unique human significance of sex stems from the fact that its full, mature functioning and fulfillment necessarily involve a relationship to persons, not to things; for the complete sexual act requires a sexually complementary "other" and, as a potentially life-transmitting process, may involve another in the person of a child. Although all relationships between persons must be governed by mutual respect, justice, and charitable concern, it should be obvious that the peculiar intimacy, interdependence, and trust necessarily involved in the sexual act, if it is to be a relationship between persons, requires the exercise of these virtues to a high degree. Thus revelation teaches and reason clearly suggests that, since sexual relations are designed both to unite the partners in a mysterious two-in-one-flesh solidarity as persons and to provide for the continuity of the race through parenthood, sex can be used responsibly only by married couples—that is, only by a man and woman who have irrevocably committed themselves to maintain an exclusive community of love and life within which they can strive for mutual happiness and fulfillment and thus create the human environment within which children can be fittingly reared.

It should be obvious that this high ideal, combining sex, love, and responsibility is not easily achieved. Men and women are not endowed with a sex instinct innately directing their sexual behavior toward clearly defined goals. Sexual relations do not automatically become expressions of love through some type of built-in or inherited necessity. As an endowment of the person, sex may be used to express a wide range of emotions and achieve a number of purposes: hate, domination, frustration, physical release, curiosity, self-display, shared enjoyment, passing affection, love, and so on. In other words, the quality of being sexed merely endows the individual with the capacity of becoming sexually mature and relating to a partner in a uniquely fulfilling, mutually responsible way.

This ideal is a goal to be achieved—a fact that underlines the need for a society to develop an adequately integrated conception of sex, in terms of which young people can gradually clarify their personal stance, and sexual standards and codes can be formulated which are consonant and supportive of mature sexuality throughout the life cycle. These codes and their associated attitudes and practices are means not ends, and consequently every generation faces the challenge of keeping them relevant to the evolving human condition.

45

HAROLD T. CHRISTENSEN

3. TOWARD A THEORY OF NORMATIVE SEXUAL MORALITY*

It is the fashion these days for popular writers to exploit the subject of sex, due to the intrinsic interest it holds. Perhaps partly as a reaction against this kind of sensational journalism, certain academicians tend to look down their noses at colleagues who deal with sex as a subject of professional interest. Nevertheless, no social scientist worth his salt is willing to be greatly influenced by either type of pressure: to jump on the bandwagon for the sake of popularity or to dodge real issues at stake in order to protect his image. Science, almost by definition, requires its workers to pursue all available data that are relevant to the solutions of their research problems, and, secondly, to keep their generalizations within the limits of their data. When the scientist goes beyond his data, as he sometimes must, it is proper that his pronouncements be labeled something like "speculations" or "interpretations."

* The author is indebted to Eugene Kanin, Hazel Kraemer, Ira Reiss, John Scott, and Athena Theodore for suggestions based upon the reading of a preliminary draft of this paper. Reprinted from the *Journal of Social Issues* 22, no. 2, 60–75.

This paper uses the scientific frame of reference to analyze the subject of sex viewed in cross-cultural perspective. Sex is a sensitive phenomenon, not only in the public view, but also as a research focus for pointing up differences across cultures. This latter fact was a major consideration in selecting it as the substantive side of a project which sought to compare normative systems.[1] The analysis to follow draws upon the writer's cross-cultural research in recent years (see reference list, items 5 through 13); but it differs from the previous articles in that this is more a discussion of issues than a formal reporting of research. It therefore attempts to interpret the generalizations in terms of dominant issues which are of social import.[2]

The concern here moves beyond sexual understanding at the descriptive level, though that too is important in its own right. The concern also transcends simple juxtaposition of the sexual cultures of several societies; as interesting as that would be, the presentation would still remain at the level of description, and, if the reader were left there, he might be tempted to ask, "so what?" Relationships among factors must be tested, most especially the relationship between behavior

[1] The project's aim was to discover evidences of how normative systems affect behavior and—what was thought even more important—affect the outcomes of behavior (see later discussion). To do this, we needed to compare some social phenomenon cross-culturally. Since sexual behavior is generally accompanied by strong feelings and sanctions, it was thought that cross-cultural differences would be greater in this than in many other areas of social action. At least a suggestion of support for this notion was found in the research itself: Premarital coitus was seen to differ cross-culturally in much greater magnitude than premarital necking; in other words, the more intimate the behavior the more accentuated the behavioral differences among normative systems (8, p. 32).

[2] Though methodological details may be found in the reports published earlier and listed at the end of this paper, the following brief description will help orient present readers. Two types of data were gathered for each of the three cultures studied (Danish, Midwest American, and Mormon American). The first was from questionnaires administered in the spring of 1958 to selected students from three universities, one from within each culture; it tapped attitudes and practices in the area of premarital sexual intimacy. The second was from record-linkage; marriage records for selected years were matched with birth and divorce records to yield data on child spacing and associated factors. Cross-cultural comparability was approached but not fully achieved, especially in the record-linkage data; identical years and lengths of search were not always maintained. Nevertheless, the cross-cultural pictures derived from these two complementary sets of data were so consistent and, in most cases, the differentials so dramatic as to lend support to the theory being tested.

and behavioral consequences and the normative systems of the societies studied. In other words, for genuine understanding one needs to move from questions of "what" to those of "how" and "why."[3]

Nevertheless, the focus here is upon the contemporary sex norms of Scandinavia and America; and even this focus is further narrowed to selected aspects of the sex norms and to the subcultures of Denmark in Scandinavia and the Midwestern region and so-called Mormon country (Utah and parts of surrounding states) in America.[4] The selection of these three subcultures for research provided a convenient range of norms and practices useful for the testing of hypotheses having both particular and general interest: particular, in seeking additional understanding of the sexual phenomenon in specified areas; general, in suggesting wider applicability of the findings and in reaching for a theory of normative systems.

DESCRIPTION OF THE NORMS

The sex norms of Denmark are known to be highly permissive; those of Midwestern United States, moderately restrictive; and those of Mormon country, highly restrictive. In Denmark—which is broadly typical of all of Scandinavia—sexual intercourse during the engagement is a tradition that

---

[3] As will be evident from the discussion to follow, we do not here mean "why" in terms of ultimate meanings or supernatural explanations, for these are beyond the reach of the scientist, but only "why" in the sense of establishing causal connections and hence finding plausible explanations within the limits of empirical data and testable relationships.

[4] In focusing upon these three subcultures, we make no pretense of describing all of the United States and Scandinavia. Nevertheless, Mormon country is known to be among the most sexually conservative sections of the United States; the Midwest, aside from being somewhat centrally located, has many bio-social characteristics that fall close to national averages; and Denmark is very much a part of Scandinavia, which, taken as a whole, manifests a considerable amount of cultural homogeneity. Concerning this last point, and with special attention to the sexual phenomenon, we should point out that our own questionnaire was administered separately to a university sample in Sweden with results remarkably similar to those of Denmark (analysis as yet unpublished). For research data on Scandinavian countries other than Denmark, and for additional evidences of sex norm homogeneity among them all, see references at the end of this paper (especially 4, 15, 17, 19, 21, 22, 23).

49

goes back three or four centuries at least, and in recent years the practice has spread to include the "going steady" relationship; now as earlier, many Danes tend to wait for pregnancy before going ahead with the wedding (1, 2, 3, 14, 15, 18, 22, 23). In the United States, including the Midwestern region—which may be taken as a fair cross-section of the whole—chastity is the code; and this prescription, though frequently violated and though undergoing considerable liberalization in recent decades, is still the dominant norm, backed heavily by a strong Judaeo-Christian tradition (16, 20). In Mormon country—which, of course, is part of the United States but, because of the particular religious culture which pervades it, is unique in many respects—chastity is a highly institutionalized norm supported by strong positive and negative sanctions. With orthodox Mormons "breaking the law of chastity" is among the most serious of sins (7, 10).

Since norms tend to be internalized within the personality structures of those who make up the society, one would expect to see cross-cultural differences, similar to those just reported, in expressions of personal attitude. This is exactly what was found. Questionnaire returns from samples of university students revealed that Danish respondents, in comparison with others:

1. Gave greater approval to both premarital coitus and postmarital infidelity (5, pp. 128–131; 12, p. 31).

2. Approved earlier starting times, in relation to marriage, of each level of intimacy—necking, petting, and coitus (12, pp. 32–35).

3. Thought in terms of a more rapid progression in intimacy development from its beginnings in necking to its completion in coitus (12, pp. 32–35).

4. Scored significantly higher on a Guttman-type scale, which combined ten separate attitudinal items into a measure of "Intimacy Permissiveness" (13, pp. 67–68).

Furthermore, since a person's behavior tends to line up with his values (including internalized norms), it follows that behavioral items can be used as indicators of the norms which lie back of them. This approach also gave support to the differing cultural patterns previously described; specifically, Danish subjects, more than others:

1. Participated in premarital coitus (13, pp. 68–69).

2. Went on to coitus from petting; that is, fewer of them engaged in terminal petting (13, p. 69, footnote 9).

3. Confined premarital coitus to one partner, and had first experience with a "steady" or fiancé (e); hence, were less promiscuous (13, p. 69. This generalization holds for males only).

4. Gave birth to an illegitimate child (7, p. 33).

5. Conceived the first legitimate child (postmarital birth) premaritally (6, p. 277; 7, p. 33; 9, p. 121).

6. Postponed further conception following the wedding; hence, showed a low proportion of early postmarital conceptions (6, p. 277; 9, pp. 121 ff.).

In virtually all of these attitudinal and behavioral measures, as well as with most others to be cited later, Mormon country fell at the opposite or restrictive end of the continuum from Denmark, with Midwestern United States in between—though closer to the Mormon than to the Danish, which is why we have labeled it "moderately restrictive."

Generally speaking, the normative system of the United States includes early, frequent, and random dating; with a gradual narrowing of the field, a gradual development of intersex intimacy, the delaying of coitus until after the wedding, and the strong expectation of marital fidelity. These patterns differ, of course, from one subgroup to another, and the Mormon segment is known to be among the strongest adherents to convention and chastity. Individual variability is great, however, and the trend over time is toward liberalization. Especially noticeable is an increase of coitus during the engagement, which is an alteration in the direction of Scandinavian practice.

The Danish system stands in sharp contrast to the American. There, dating (which is a relatively recent innovation)

51

starts later, is less widely practiced, and is more likely to begin with a "going steady" arrangement and an expectation of marriage to follow. Furthermore, all levels of sexual intimacy are accepted once the relationship becomes firmly established; and the progression to complete intimacy is relatively rapid. As a matter of fact, the Danes do not draw a sharp line to set off technical chastity (as do Americans) but rather regard petting and coitus as belonging together and see them both as appropriate in a relationship based on love and oriented toward marriage. Today, this kind of a relationship is most apt to be established with "going steady" in Denmark but not until the engagement in America (cf. 12, p. 31). Actually, in Denmark both "going steady" and engagement mean more in terms of commitment and privileges than they do in America, and the wedding probably means less—relatively speaking. It is to be noted, therefore, that the greater sexual permissiveness in Denmark (and all of Scandinavia for that matter) does not necessarily imply greater looseness or higher promiscuity; intimacy is simply made more a part of the courting and marrying processes. Nevertheless, it must be additionally observed that there seems to have been a spreading or generalizing of this marriage-oriented permissiveness to nonmarital situations, for the Danes gave greater approval to all of our propositions regarding intimacy (12, pp. 31–35) and also showed higher rates of illegitimacy (7, p. 33). Finally, though the trend in recent years is toward the adoption of American dating patterns, and though the cultures on both sides of the Atlantic are moving toward convergence, differences in sex norms are still striking enough to give illumination to certain vital issues.

ANALYSIS OF THE ISSUES

Attention is now turned to four basic questions which pinpoint major issues in the sex problem that can be approached via cross-cultural research. Since the majority of readers will be American, the questions are phrased in terms of effects of restrictiveness.

1. How does restrictiveness affect deviation from the norm?

Norms have been taken to mean the prescriptions or rules of conduct that a society imposes upon its members, whether formally or informally. They are reflected in the verbalizations and overt behavior of the people. Nevertheless, though behavior may be taken as an index of a norm, it is not the norm itself, and, most importantly, it will usually vary somewhat from the norm. Rarely, if ever, is the fit between prescription and performance a perfect one. Yet discrepancies of this sort lead to tension and disorganization in the systems involved.

As has been seen, the performance measures of sexual behavior did tend to line up broadly with expectation within each of the three normative systems, though this told us nothing of specific deviations. To get at the latter, we compared within each culture the percentage of those who approved premarital coitus with the percentage who actually had experienced it (13, pp. 70–72). Here are the results:

1. For Denmark, substantially more approved than had had experience.

2. For the two American samples, the reverse was true: substantially more had had experience than approved.

3. Of the American samples, this discrepancy between experience and approval was greater for Mormon country.

Explanation for the Danish pattern probably lies in the permissive norms of that culture, coupled with the youthfulness and hence lack of marriage orientation of many of the respondents. (Recall that premarital intercourse in Denmark is more frequently tied in with love and commitment to marry; many hadn't yet reached that stage, though they approved of coitus for those who had.) Explanation for the American patterns, and most especially that of Mormon country, probably lies in the restrictiveness of the culture, coupled with biological and social pressures upon individuals to violate the norms.

53

But whatever the explanations, the conclusion that norm violation varies directly with norm restrictiveness seems almost inescapable.

Yet, it must be emphasized that we are now speaking of deviation from internalized norms—the case in which the individual violates his own standards. The suggestion that this kind of norm violation is proportionately greater in restrictive societies in no sense contradicts the earlier conclusion that societies with restrictive norms also have higher proportions showing restrictive behavior; United States in contrast to Denmark, and Mormon country in contrast to the Midwest, were disproportionately high in both respects. Thus it can be said, tentatively at least, that sex norm restrictiveness elicits greater conformity to the prescribed goal (for example, chastity) than does sex norm permissiveness but at the same time results in greater nonconformity assimilated to the value structure of the people: the relationship specified will be relative to whether one is thinking of a nominal category (first instance) or an internalized value system (second instance).

2. How does restrictiveness affect the consequences of norm deviation?

Even more important to our theory than deviation from norms is the question of consequences. We are interested in knowing the effects of norm violation and how these compare across cultures. Following are some summary points taken from the research:

1. Of the males and females who had experienced premarital coitus, proportionately more from Mormon country did so out of coercion and/or felt obligation, and experienced guilt and other negative feelings subsequent to the event. Danish respondents were lowest on these reactions (13, pp. 69–70).

2. Of those who became premaritally pregnant, the tendency in Mormon country was to marry even before confirming the pregnancy; in the Midwest, to marry immediately after the pregnancy was definitely known,

or about two months after conception; and in Denmark, to not let pregnancy pressure them into hurrying the wedding—most of these Danish marriages took place about five months after conception (6, pp. 275–278; 7, pp. 35–36).

3. Percentage differences by which divorce rates in the premarital exceeded those in the postmarital pregnancy groups were highest in Mormon country and lowest in Denmark (6, p. 278; 7, pp. 36–38; 9, pp. 123–126).

Admittedly these three measures of consequences do not exhaust the possibilities; yet they deal with crucial points and at least suggest what the outcome of a more comprehensive analysis might be.[5] Here it is seen that the most permissive culture (Denmark) shows the least negative effects from both premarital coitus and premarital pregnancy: guilt and kindred feelings are at a minimum; there is little pressure to advance the wedding date; and the influence of these intimacies upon subsequent divorce is relatively small. Conversely, negative effects are in each instance greater in the most restrictive culture (Mormon country), with the more moderate culture (Midwestern) showing in-between effects.

It would seem that the negative consequences[6] of norm deviation tend to vary directly with norm restrictiveness—probably because deviation in the more restrictive societies represents a larger gap between norms and behavior and, hence, constitutes a greater offense.

---

[5] In the writer's research, an additional cross-cultural comparison of consequences attempted to get the relative effects of early postmarital conception. When divorce rates for "early postmarital conceivers" were compared with those of "normal postmarital conceivers" the differential was lowest (in fact, almost nonexistent) for Mormon country—which is according to expectation under our theory, since in that culture early postmarital conception is the norm. In the other two cultures, where the practice is more to delay the starting of the family, early postmarital conception was found to be associated with higher than average divorce rates (9, Tables 2 and 3).

[6] Though we use the terms "effects" and "consequences," it is recognized that association is not the same thing as causation and that the latter has not actually been established. It is possible, for example, that with reference to divorce rate differentials (point 3 above) a selective process is operating, which, in the restrictive Mormon culture could throw disproportionately more divorce-prone individuals into the premarital pregnancy category—if it should be that premarital pregnancy proneness and divorce proneness are linked

3. How does restrictiveness affect patterns of subcultural variation?

In building normative theory, it would be important to know if there is any relationship between the strength of norms and the homogeneity of culture. The following findings from the author's research are relevant to this question.

1. The two extremes on our permissiveness-restrictiveness continuum, that is, Denmark and Mormon country, showed the greatest convergence of male and female attitudes. Furthermore, proportionately more respondents from these cultures, and especially from the Danish, believed in a single standard of sexual morality (5, pp. 129–132, 134–137; 12, p. 32; 13, p. 74).

2. When it comes to behavior, however, only the permissive culture (Denmark) showed a strong convergence of male and female patterns.[7] As a matter of fact, the most restrictive (Mormon country) tended to be the most divergent in this respect—a fact which, when combined with attitudinal homogeneity between the sexes, means, as pointed out earlier, that disproportionately large numbers there fail to practice what they profess (5, p. 135, footnote 2; 13, pp. 68–74).

3. An incomplete testing[8] of cross-cultural differences in homogeneity of sex attitudes according to certain other variables—age, education, residence, social class, church attendance, and so forth—revealed Mormon country with the fewest and Denmark with the most intrafactor significant differences. For example, high versus low

within the personality—for the presumption is that cultural restrictiveness would tend to eliminate from premarital pregnancy those whose personalities are more conforming. The matter needs further study. Nevertheless, we would hypothesize that selectivity, if it exists, would account for only part of the explanation; that an important remainder would be causal.

[7] There is still a further evidence that permissiveness makes for homogeneity at the behavioral level: Just as the most permissive of the cultures (Denmark) showed the smallest male-female difference, so the more permissive of the sexes (males) showed the smallest cross-cultural differences in premarital coitus (13, p. 68, Table 2).

[8] So far the tests have been confined to attitudes toward marital infidelity and have not included attitudes toward premarital practices or any of the behavior patterns.

church attendance differentiated attitudes toward marital infidelity in a statistically significant way in Denmark, but not in Mormon country (5, pp. 132–137).

Though explanations are not clearly visible within the data, there are some which seem plausible. As to attitude, we would hypothesize that the male-female convergence in Denmark is due to a freeing or liberalizing of the female, whereas in Mormon country it is due to a taming or conventionalizing of the male—through stress on authority, conformity, and participation within the church, all of which are reinforced by a lay priesthood involving most male members twelve years of age and over. As to behavior, we would hazard the guess that in Denmark, where there is little stigma attached to pre-marital sex activity, behavior tends to follow the norms, and hence male-female similarity in attitude becomes male-female similarity in behavior also; whereas, in Mormon country, where the standards set by the church may be somewhat utopian in nature, a stronger sex urge among males,[9] plus a persuasive double standard in the general culture, causes more males than females to violate the norms, which in turn increases the gap by which the two sexes diverge. As to the third finding, which describes the prominence of certain other subcategories as differing across our three normative systems, we would tentatively suggest the following: In permissive Denmark, sexual codes are more flexible and the resulting wider range of tolerance permits greater development of the subgroups; whereas, in restrictive America, and especially in Mormon country, there is a greater rigidity of the codes and a narrower range of tolerance, which discourage deviation and the development of subgroups and subcultures.

4. Can sex norms and their consequences be generalized across cultures?

Science looks for uniformities in nature; out of analysis comes synthesis and general theory. In the spirit of science,

---

[9] Though the existence of male-female differences in biological sex drive is open to some question and is in need of further research, there can be little doubt but that in our culture most males have stronger learned sexual desire than do females.

sociology and kindred disciplines search for principles of human behavior that can be generalized over time and across cultures. But the social sciences also see the peculiarities of each culture and, recognizing this, tend to adhere to a theory of cultural relativism. In the preceding pages we have observed ways in which sexual attitudes and behaviors and behavior consequences are relative to cultural norms. Nevertheless, not everything is relative. Here are some phenomena in our research which were found to apply to each of the three cultures studied—though not always in the same degree:

1. Most sexual intimacy and reproductive pregnancy occur within the institutional bounds of marriage.

2. The modal timing of first postmarital conception is approximately one month after the wedding (6, p. 273).

3. Patterns of sexual behavior are strongly correlated with personal attitudes and social norms; permissive thinking tends to beget permissive behavior and restrictive thinking, restrictive behavior (13, pp. 70–71).

4. Approval of nonmarital coitus, as applied to the premarital period, increases with each specified advance in involvement and/or commitment between the couple; but, as applied to the postmarital period, the reverse is true (5, pp. 130–131; 12, p. 31).

5. Females are more conservative in sexual matters than are males, almost without exception and regardless of the measure used or whether it measures attitudes or behavior (5, pp. 131–132; 12, pp. 31–35; 13, pp. 68–72).

6. Females who engage in premarital coitus are more likely than males to do so because of pressure or felt obligation, and are also more likely than males to have as a partner either a "steady" or a fiancé(e) (13, p. 70).

7. There is a suggestion—though the testing was inconclusive—that persons who have premarital coitus are disproportionately low on satisfaction derived from their courtships (13, pp. 72–73).

8. Premaritally pregnant couples subsequently experience

higher divorce rates than the postmaritally pregnant (6, p. 276; 9, pp. 123–126).

9. Of the premarital pregnancy couples, higher divorce rates are found for the "shotgun" type, that is, those who wait for marriage until just before the child is born, than for those who marry soon after pregnancy (7, p. 39; 9, pp. 123–126).

10. Of the postmarital pregnancy couples, higher divorce rates are found for the early conceivers than for those who wait a few months before starting their families (6, p. 276; 9, pp. 126–127).

11. Premarital pregnancy is greater among young brides and grooms in contrast to older ones, among those who have a civil wedding in contrast to a religious one, and among those in a laboring line of work in contrast to the more skilled and professional occupations (6, pp. 274–275; 7, pp. 34–35; 8, pp. 39–40; 9, p. 121).

To repeat, each of the above statements is applicable to all three of the cultures studied: Danish, Midwestern and Mormon country. Though these items do not apply in equal strength to each of the samples, they do represent significant regularities that can be generalized.

Toward a Theory of Normative Morality

The term morality is used commonly to designate conduct that is considered "good" or "right," frequently conceived in terms of absolutes.[10] But questions of ultimates and absolutes lie outside the reach of science, and the best the scientist can do with them—in fact, all he can do as scientist—is to maintain suspended judgment and apply objective analysis. Assertion without evidence is the essence of dogmatism, and the scientist as well as the religionist can be dogmatic, though to do so puts him beyond his data.

---

[10] Though morality is popularly thought of in terms of absolute guidelines based upon eternal truths, this is not the only definitional possibility. As used here, the term encompasses any system of "right" and "wrong," whether it be based upon transcendental notions or empirical observations.

59

What, then, can science add to the field of morals; and, if anything, at what points can it contribute? Can there be a sociological basis for decisions on proper behavior? If by "proper" is meant something that is intrinsically or eternally right, the answer to this last question is "no," but if the meaning is simply that the behavior lines up with group norms, and hence escapes the consequences of negative group sanctions, the answer is "yes." Though the sociologist cannot decide what is best in an absolute sense, he can determine what is most functional to the systems involved[11]—and hence help decide what is best in a relative sense.

It should be evident, then, that the task of the scientist is not to actually set up or affirm a moral system, not, in other words, to take a moral position—even one based upon empirical evidence—but only to determine cause and effect relationships which can aid the nonscientist (including the scientist in his nonscientist role as a citizen) in choosing criteria for moral decision. The scientist, being confined to empirical data, cannot touch questions of absolutistic morality; nor can he, while in his professional role, make choices among the alternatives of relativistic (normative) morality. But he can clarify the alternatives and thus contribute something to moral questions.

Normative morality is defined here as any code of right and wrong that is founded upon the operations of normative systems. It is more, however, than the particular systems standing by themselves; for only by knowing the ways in which these interrelate, how personal behaviors deviate from social prescriptions, and what the consequences of such deviations are, can there be any rational basis for moral decision. Thus normative morality is relativistic rather than absolutistic. It attempts to put science in place of polemics and to see

11 According to the structural-functional school, human activities tend to become organized into intra- and interdependent systems, which perpetuate themselves only by maintaining necessary degrees of balance or equilibrium. There are personality systems and social systems—and subsystems of each—all interrelated. When an activity is in harmony with and helps to maintain a system it is said to be functional; when the reverse is true, dysfunctional.

It is thus possible to use system maintenance as the criterion against which the propriety of behavior is decided. This, essentially, is what we mean by a normative morality.

questions of right and wrong in terms of the measurable and variable consequences of the behavior involved. At this stage of inquiry, we can only speak of moving toward such a theory, for the crucial hypotheses are only now being formulated and their testing is as yet but meager and exploratory.

Though the social scientist, as scientist, cannot make value judgments, he is entitled to study values as data. As a matter of fact, this is more than his privilege; it is his obligation. The values people hold tend both to shape their behavior and to determine the effects of this behavior upon themselves, upon others, and upon society at large. Values are intervening variables which, for any genuine understanding, must be taken into account.

One small attempt at preliminary testing and theory formulation is the cross-cultural research summarized here. This has focused upon the sex side of the question—with the realization, of course, that morality is concerned with more than sexual behavior, but, also, with the accompanying belief than any increased understanding of even a small part of a phenomenon is likely to give some illumination to the whole.[12] In the following concluding paragraphs let us further speculate as to what may have been accomplished and what the next steps might be.

We have demonstrated for the three cultures studied that sex patterns show both regularities and variabilities. If everything were regular—that is, generalizable across cultures—one could look to these universals as bases for a uniform morality;[13] or, if everything were culture-bound, one could con-

---

[12] It is also realized that present generalizations are based upon samples from a very limited number of cultures and that even within these samples the phenomenon has been only preliminarily explored. Furthermore, not all of the summary points given in this paper were found to have statistical significance. (For details on this and other matters, the reader is referred to the original publications given in the reference list.) Nevertheless, it is felt that the findings are sufficiently reasonable and consistent to provide guidelines for future research and theory building.

[13] Even if it could be demonstrated that the consequences of given sex acts are the same everywhere and at all times (which it cannot), the scientist still could not conclude that these effects are absolute, with implications of transcendental meaning—for he is bound to the study of empirical data. The scientist is within his sphere studying questions of universality, but this is as close as he can permit himself to come to questions of absolute or ultimate morality.

clude that nothing is fixed and morality is entirely relative. The truth of the matter seems to lie between these two conditions.

Many of the regularities found (suggestive of universals) seem to be the kinds of things one would expect to be functional to personality systems and/or social systems per se: confining reproduction, for the most part, to marriage; maintaining a reasonable alignment between beliefs and practices; females being more conservative regarding sex beliefs and practices than males; divorce being greater than average among the premaritally pregnant, and especially among those of the "shotgun marriage" variety; et cetera.

Logical explanations for these regularities are not difficult to find. To give but two brief examples: (1) Females everywhere tend to be more conservative in sexual matters than males because by nature they are tied more closely to the reproductive process, which, disproportionally for them, increases the hazards of unprotected intimacy (men can't get pregnant) and also because most cultures hold a double standard which places the female offender under greater social condemnation. (2) Premarital pregnancy is regularly associated with disproportionately high divorce rates, both because some divorce-prone individuals are pressured into marriage, though love and/or adequate preparation may be lacking, and because in all cultures (though more in certain ones than others) there will be some of the premaritally pregnant who will harbor feelings of guilt or blame which can frustrate their personalities and disrupt their relationships. In other words, the explanations seem to lie in both selection and causation, and we would hypothesize that both of these operate to some extent in all cultures. If space permitted, it would be possible to extend these arguments and also to speculate concerning other factors. Nevertheless, for any general theory of morality based upon the regularity of consequences, it will be necessary to go beyond logic and to carry out research on these and related points.

But a general morality may not be possible—at least not without severe qualification—simply because the consequences of sexual acts are not always the same; they differ in degree if not in kind, depending upon the cultural milieu in which they occur. For example, regarding the case of pre-marital pregnancy and divorce just cited, though the relation-ship between these two factors was regular (in the same direction) in all three of the cultures studied, it was also rela-tive to each culture: Divorce rate differentials between pre-marital and postmarital conceivers were lowest in Denmark and highest in Mormon country, suggesting that negative effects vary directly with the restrictiveness of the normative system.

A relativistic (normative) sexual morality would judge acts in terms of their varying consequences. In the research dealt with here, we have found for the premaritally intimate in Mormon country (the most restrictive of the samples) not only higher divorce rate differentials but also greater guilt and a stronger tendency to seek escape from conscience and social condemnation by hurrying up the wedding. Two addi-tional items pertaining to Mormon culture seem relevant at this point. First, of the three cultures studied, this one showed the highest percentage of respondents engaging in terminal petting, which suggests that its very strict proscription against premarital coitus may be resulting in an excess of precoital activity carried out for its own sake; at least there seems to be a tendency there, more than in the other cultures and especially the Danish, to draw the line separating moral from immoral sexual behavior just short of chastity. The second item to be mentioned (though not part of the research pre-viously cited in this paper) is that age at marriage shows up as disproportionately low in Mormon country; as a matter of fact, in recent years Utah has been among the highest of the reporting states in percentage of teen-age marriages (11, pp. 29, 33, footnote 6). Explanations for this cultural differ-ence probably lie in the severity of the religious sanctions in support of the chastity norm, plus heavy romantic-sexual stimulants in the general culture, reinforced by church teach-ing on the importance and sacredness of marriage and church programs bringing young people together at early ages and somewhat continuously—plus the petting pattern just noted. All of this would seem to leave boys and girls charged emotionally and/or stimulated sexually, yet without socially approved modes of release except marriage. But the matter needs to be researched.

We have used Morman culture in our analysis in order to accentuate the contrasts. It must be kept in mind, however, that the average or more typical American culture has these same differences compared with Scandinavia, though to a lesser degree, and the explanations might be expected to be similar: The United States has more terminal petting, younger ages at marriage, more guilt associated with premarital coitus, a greater tendency to hurry the wedding when caught with pregnancy, a disproportionately higher divorce rate associated with premarital pregnancy, and so on. Some of the writer's Danish acquaintances have, in defense of their system, even gone further than these research points and suggested that the restrictiveness of American culture—including its emphasis upon technical chastity while at the same time permitting petting—is resulting in larger proportions of such "pathologies" as cheesecake publications, hardcore pornography, prostitution, and homosexuality. Whether or not these asserted differences would hold up under research remains to be seen; they do make interesting hypotheses.

What, then, can be said about the relative merits of the Scandinavian and American sexual systems? Certainly nothing by way of ultimate judgment (unless one abandons science and accepts the tenets of transcendental morality). Seen in terms of behavioral consequences, which is the view of normative morality, there are both functional and dysfunctional practices within both cultures—some of which have been outlined above. But when a thing is recognized as dysfunctional, this judgment is only with reference to the normative system in which it exists; and whether, in order to obtain equilibrium, one should change the behavior to fit the system, or the system to fit the behavior, or some of both, is a question for the religionist or the philosopher, not the scientist.

In recent years, American sexual practices have been moving in the direction of the more liberal Scandinavian norms. Some people argue that this will be the solution to our problems. It must be remembered, however, that consequences are relative to the systems within which the behavior takes place. The functionality or dysfunctionality of American sex practices must be seen against American sex norms, and unless the latter have been liberalizing as rapidly as the former there will have been an increase of strains (dysfunctions) within the personalities and the relationships involved. There is at least a suggestion that this may be happening. It could be, for example, that the increasing rates of personal and marital disorganization of recent decades are due in part to an enlarging sex freedom in the face of a lagging sex ethics. But whether or not the gap separating prescription from practice actually is getting larger, at least it exists, and its existence calls for objective investigation and analysis—as background for decision and adjustment.

Within the framework of normative morality, an act is "good" if it succeeds and "bad" if it fails in terms of meaningful criteria. For the scientist, the most meaningful criterion appropriate to moral judgment is the action's nearness of fit to the values or norms which govern the behavior. There has been little research relating nonmarital sexual behavior to its measurable consequences, which may be presumed to exist. Of the existing objective studies (as well as causal speculations) on this problem, some have been solely concerned with possible effects upon the individual, his mental health and adjustments; others with possible effects upon the pair relationship, whether it is made mutually reinforcing or enduring; and still others upon possible effects upon the community or society, whether there are interconnections between sexual controls and societal stability. It is our contention that a theory of normative morality, if it is to be built, must draw upon culturally relevant research relating to all of these effect levels.

REFERENCES

1. Anderson, Robert T., and Anderson, Gallatin. "Sexual Behavior and Urbanization in a Danish Village." *Southwestern Journal of Anthropology* 16 (1960) 93–109.
2. Auken, Kirsten. "Time of Marriage, Mate Selection and Task

Accomplishment in Newly Formed Copenhagen Families." *Acta Sociologica* 8 (1964) 138–41.

3. ———. *Unge Kvinders Sexuelle Adfaerd.* Copenhagen: Rosenkilds og Bagger, 1953. English summary, pp. 389–402.

4. Birgitta, Linner. *Society and Sex in Sweden.* Stockholm: Swedish Institute for Cultural Relations, 1955. Pamphlet, 37 pp.

5. Christensen, Harold T. "A Cross-cultural Comparison of Attitudes Toward Marital Infidelity." *International Journal of Comparative Sociology* 3 (1962) 124–37.

6. ———. "Child Spacing Analysis via Record Linkage: New Data Plus a Summing up from Earlier Reports." *Marriage and Family Living* 25 (1963) 272–80.

7. ———. "Cultural Relativism and Premarital Sex Norms." *American Sociological Review* 25 (1960) 31–39.

8. ———. "Selected Aspects of Child Spacing in Denmark." *Acta Sociologica* 4 (1959) 35–45.

9. ———. "Timing of First Pregnancy as a Factor in Divorce: A Cross-cultural Analysis." *Eugenics Quarterly* 10 (1963) 119–30.

10. ———. "Value Variables in Pregnancy Timing: Some Intercultural Comparisons." In N. Anderson, ed., *Studies of the Family,* vol. 3. Gottingen: Vandenhoech & Ruprecht, 1958. Pp. 29–45.

11. Christensen, Harold T., and Cannon, Kenneth L. "Temple versus Non-temple Marriage in Utah: Some Demographic Considerations." *Social Science* 39 (1964) 26–33.

12. Christensen, Harold T., and Carpenter, George R. "Timing Patterns in the Development of Sexual Intimacy." *Marriage and Family Living* 24 (1962) 30–35.

13. ———. "Value-Behavior Discrepancies Regarding Premarital Coitus in Three Western Cultures." *American Sociological Review* 27 (1962) 66–74.

14. Croog, Sydney H. "Aspects of the Cultural Background of Premarital Pregnancy in Denmark." *Social Forces* 30 (1951) 215–19.

15. ———. "Premarital Pregnancies in Scandinavia and Finland." *American Journal of Sociology* 57 (1962) 358–65.

16. Ehrmann, Winston. "Marital and Nonmarital Sexual Be-

havior." In H. T. Christensen, ed., *Handbook of Marriage and the Family.* Chicago: Rand McNally, 1964. Pp. 585–622.

17. Eliot, Thomas D., *et al. Norway's Families: Trends, Problems, Programs.* Philadelphia: University of Philadelphia Press, 1960.

18. Hansen, George. *Saedelighedsforhold Blandt Landbeforkningen i Denmark i det 18 Aarhundrede.* Copenhagen: Det Danske Forlag, 1957.

19. Jonsson, Gustav. "Sexualvanor hos Svensk Ungdom." In *Ungdomen Moter Samhallet.* Stockholm: K. L. Beckmans Boktyckeri, 1951. Pp. 160–204.

20. Reiss, Ira L. *Premarital Sexual Standards in America.* Glencoe, Ill.: Free Press, 1960.

21. Sturup, Georg K. "Sex Offenses: The Scandinavian Experience." *Law and Contemporary Problems* 25 (1960) 361–75.

22. Svalastoga, Kaare. "The Family in Scandinavia." *Marriage and Family Living* 16 (1954) 374–80.

23. Wikman, K. Robert. *Die Einleitung der Ehe.* Aabo, Finland: Acta Academiae Aaboensis, 1937, XI.

JOSEPH B. TAMNEY

4. FAMILY SOLIDARITY AND FERTILITY

The explanation of fertility is obviously not a constant. Family size reflects the total situation in which people find themselves. Today we postulate an approaching decline in fertility because of the increasing availability of birth control methods and the economic needs of the world population. But will economic considerations maintain their tyranny over fertility? Robert Heilbroner recently predicted "that the general dimensions of the problem make it possible to envisage the substantial alleviation—perhaps even the virtual elimination—of massive poverty within the limits of capitalism three or four decades hence, or possibly even sooner."[1]

This decline in the significance of economic factors seems part of a more general trend that will see most of the hardship taken out of childbearing and rearing. For instance,

---

[1] Robert L. Heilbroner, "The Future of Capitalism," *Commentary* 41, no. 4 (April 1966) 26. More specifically, he writes, "If the trend of growth of the past century is continued, the average level of real wages for industrial labor should double in another two or three decades. This would bring average earnings to a level of about $10,000 and would effectively spell the abolition of wage poverty, under any definition" (p. 25).

increasing affluence will be accompanied by greater availability of child care services. In this regard Russia seems to be leading the way; it is estimated that by the end of the year half of the urban preprimary-school population will be in some type of day care center.[2] In this country pressure for similar services is coming from three sources: those who are concerned with helping poor people become self-supporting, middle and upper class women eager to give their sex the same opportunities now reserved for men, and child specialists who believe in the educational benefits such services would offer children:

> Day care is not a substitute for any other service; it has unique values of its own. Can we agree, then, that it is time day care asserted these values for all children and stopped feeling guilty because it permitted a child to be separated from his mother? Can we not go even further and proclaim that day care can offer something valuable to children *because* they are separated from their parents?
>
> Frankly, what we have to offer children could not be given them if they remained at home. We can provide them with enriched programs, with thoughtful and skilled personnel, with settings in which they are free to play actively, and even with freedom from their mothers for part of the day. Where else can young children gain so much?[3]

The combination of this positive ideology and the political pressures being exerted by the aforementioned groups suggests that, in the not too distant future, day care facilities will be as prevalent here as they will be in Russia—though they might be of a different type.

The significance of this development seems twofold: (1) it will diminish the importance of some of the traditional arguments for a large family, namely those which have centered on the benefits to the children of being raised with a large number of siblings. For instance, people argue that this forces the children to develop a sense of cooperativeness, but obviously such would result from participation in a day care

---

[2] Peter Juviler, "Soviet Families," *Survey* 60 (July 1966) 56.
[3] Milton Willner, "Day Care: A Reassessment," *Child Welfare* 44, no. 3 (March 1965) 129–30.

center. In a way such facilities will mean that every child will grow up "in a large family." And (2) the combination of affluence and aid in caring for children will severely lessen the punishments associated with having children. Rainwater believes that there is one central norm governing family size decisions in our society: "One shouldn't have more children than one can support, but one should have as many children as one can afford."[4] Given the changes we have discussed, and this norm, the future would seem to be a time of large families.[5]

The question arises, therefore: Are there any forces that will counteract this tendency? One, of course, is the threat of overpopulation, and this will no doubt be an important one. Yet it is a somewhat vague pressure; everyone can agree that the world should not be overpopulated, and yet not be at all clear as to what that means in terms of how many children he or she should have.

In discussing the widespread significance of economic factors in lowering family size, Berelson wrote: "The very circumstances of life have produced what may be called a natural motivation toward family planning as distinguishable from the contrived motivation that may result from the informational campaigns if perceived as artificial—and the former are far more desirable and consequential than the latter."[6] The argument from overpopulation might indeed be artificial and less than effective. The purpose of this paper is to explore the possibility that new "natural" forces might be developing which would limit family size in a time of affluence and child care facilities; we shall do this from the per-

---

[4] Lee Rainwater, *Family Design: Marital Sexuality, Family Size, and Contraception* (Chicago: Aldine, 1965) 150.

[5] Signs of such a change seem to exist already: "In both 1941 and 1945, approximately nine-tenths of the respondents reported an ideal of two, three, or four children—about the same proportion as in our 1955 and 1960 GAF studies. Within this range, however, the most popular number shifted from two in 1941 to three in 1945 and then to four in 1955 and 1960, and the average increased from 3.0 to 3.5." Pascal K. Whelpton *et al.*, *Fertility and Family Planning in the United States* (Princeton, N.J.: Princeton University Press, 1966) 34.

[6] Bernard Berelson, "KAP Studies in Fertility" in Bernard Berelson *et al.*, eds., *Family Planning and Population Programs* (Chicago: University of Chicago Press, 1966) 660.

spective of solidarity. The following section discusses the meaning of and conditions for solidarity. The final section will consider the rewards of family solidarity and the possible effects of contemporary social changes on such solidarity.

THE REALITY OF SOCIAL AGGREGATES

There exists a continuum of involvement which is applicable to all relations. Any two units are more or less involved with each other, that is, more or less the same thing.[7] Leibniz seems to have realized both the fact that all things are more or less the same thing and that no true social unit exists:

> The conception of substance necessarily implies the idea of unity. No one thinks that two stones very far apart form a single substance. If now we imagine them joined and soldered together, will this juxtaposition change the nature of things? Of course not; this will be two stones and not a single one. If now we imagine them attached by an irresistible force, the impossibility of separating them will not prevent the mind from distinguishing them and will not prevent their remaining two and not one. In a word every compound is no more a single substance than is a pile of sand or a sack of wheat. We might as well say that the employees of the India Company formed a single substance.[8]

Every social aggregate is a compound, and therefore not a unit; on the other hand, some aggregates are more a unit than others. Sociologists have spent too much time arguing whether a group is real. We suggest that the important question is the empirical one: how real is a particular aggregate? In this paper we equate social solidarity with social reality

---

[7] R. T. Ladd wrote: "Every relation appears . . . as a partial unification of two beings." Quoted in Funk and Wagnall's *New Standard Dictionary*, 1952, from: R. T. Ladd, *A Theory of Reality*. And Aristotle wrote that the good man "is related to his friend as to himself (for his friend is another self)." Richard McKeon, ed., *Introduction to Aristotle* (New York: Modern Library, 1947) 502.

[8] Paul Janet, "Introduction" in *Leibniz: Discourse on Metaphysics, and Correspondence with Arnauld, and Monodology* (La Salle, Ill.: Open Court, 1962) xiv.

and will discuss variables which seem to determine the extent to which an aggregate is experienced as real.

Human beings live in a perceptual world, that is, there are laws of perception which organize or solidify our field of experience. "Elements in experience are automatically and almost irresistibly grouped—other things equal—according to proximity, similarity and continuity."[9] The first two criteria are especially important for sociology; they mean that we perceive people who are close together as forming a group, as well as those who are physically similar, such as people with the same skin color. It must be emphasized that even before we begin to think about people, or before we know whether individuals belong to the same club or work for the same company, we organize our social fields according to purely perceptual criteria. Hilgard has stressed the significance of this for social interaction:

> We group together those of similar appearance, clothing, or mannerisms, assuming more congeniality, perhaps, than the similarity assures; we tend to see those who live near together or who associate together as sharing common values or beliefs (including "guilt by association"); we structure the social environment into figure and ground as we do the impersonal environment. When a figure appears, the boundaries are sharpened, and the distinction between what belongs to the figure and what belongs to the ground becomes clear; we may thus structure the world into the "free world" and the "communist world," ignoring many of the other differences between nations and governments.[10]

The significant point is that before we "find out" about the social organization of an aggregate, if we have visually encountered them, we have already organized this aggregate according to the laws of perception. Things are more or less real, they are more or less perceptually one, depending on the extent to which they are close, similar and continuous. *A social aggregate is experienced as real, therefore, to the*

[9] Bernard Berelson and Gary A. Steiner, *Human Behavior* (New York: Harcourt, 1964) 106.

[10] Ernest R. Hilgard, *Introduction to Psychology*, 3rd ed. (New York: Harcourt, 1962) 552–53.

extent that the members of an aggregate have been solidified perceptually.[11]

As Jerome Bruner notes, a key function of language is that it helps us overcome these perceptual laws.[12] Language allows us to regroup objects in the field of experience; it permits us to organize objects we do not even perceive. It is one of the contentions of this paper that this does not eliminate our awareness of perceptual organizations, but means that human beings are capable of two different types of organizations: perceptual and cognitive. This leads us to our second princip'e concerning social solidarity: *The extent to which an aggregate is experienced as real depends on the degree of overlap between the perceptual and cognitive organizations of the field.*

Although it is not possible to presently prove this principle, some illustrative evidence might at least suggest its importance. Carpenter has written that: "An important clue to social relations in primate societies is the observed spatial relations of individuals, sub-groups, and organized groups. The strength of the attachment between two individuals may be judged, or actually measured by observing for a period of time the average distance which separates the two animals."[13]

---

[11] It must be kept in mind, however, that these laws of perception are not equally applicable at all times and places. "The classical Gestalt laws of visual organization . . . are often presented as unchanging; yet the laws of proximity, similarity, common fate, and so on, as known in adults may change progressively with age. Rush studied children and adolescents between about six and twenty-two years of age (the first grade through college). She presented simple dot patterns which could be organized in one or more ways and determined which method of visual organization was dominant. Her results cast doubt upon the 'unchanging' nature of visual organization, since the efficacy of continuity, similarity, proximity, and direction as principles change with age. Continuity of patterns increases in efficacy up to about fourteen years of age and then drops off to a lower level. Similarity and proximity both steadily increase in efficacy with age. And there is a shift from seeing equally spaced dot patterns as rows to seeing them as columns—a shift from horizontal to vertical emphasis in visual organization." (Reference is to: Grace Rush, "Visual Grouping in Relation to Age," *Archives of Psychology* 31, no. 217 [1937–38] 95.) Charles M. Solley and Gardner Murphy, *Development of the Perceptual World* (New York: Basic Books, 1960) 142.

[12] Jerome S. Bruner, ed., *Studies in Cognitive Growth* (New York: John Wiley, 1966).

[13] C. R. Carpenter, "Societies of Monkeys and Apes," in Charles Southwick, ed., *Primate Social Behavior* (Princeton, N.J.: Van Nostrand, 1963) 36.

Similarly Ardrey stresses the congruity between spatial arrangements and power relations among various species.[14] Λ. D. Bain reversed dominance relations by changing spatial relations among the great tit.[15] In general, vertebrates have maintained congruence between physical proximity and social relatedness. It would seem hazardous to avoid the possibility that this overlapping between perceptual and cognitive fields might not also be important for homo sapiens.

Moreover, man has acknowledged the continued importance of the principles governing perceptual organization. The stress on blood, for instance, illustrates the continued significance of the spatial or proximity principle. Observers of the 1965 riots in Watts, a Negro section of Los Angeles, described the following scene: "As they passed a small gas station, several people wanted to set it afire. One of the people standing nearby the station told them: 'Let it stand. Blood owns it.' "[16] Blood relationship seems to imply that at one time in the past, two objects participated in the same mother object. The reference might be to a time far back in history, but blood similarity seems to imply perceptually based identity with a common object. The continued importance of "blood" in our society illustrates the continued significance of a sense of spatial oneness, and thus of the perceptual organization of our experience.

Heberle has noted that in at least parts of rural Germany, neighbors, people physically close, had precedence over friends in the celebration of family rituals.[17] This again affirms the significance of proximity. Given the importance of cognitive organization and this evidence illustrating that perceptual principles do affect human behavior, it does not seem farfetched to hypothesize that the experience of solidarity depends in part on the degree of overlap between the perceptual and cognitive organizations of our experience.

[14] Robert Ardrey, "The Drive for Territory," *Life,* August 26, 1966, p. 46.

[15] Edward T. Hall, *The Hidden Dimension* (Garden City, N.Y.: Doubleday, 1966) 9.

[16] Jerry Cohen and William S. Murphy, *Burn, Baby, Burn* (New York: Dutton, 1966) 111.

[17] Rudolph Heberle, "The Normative Element in Neighborhood Relations," *Pacific Sociological Review* 3, no. 1 (Spring 1960) 4.

Until this point we have simply referred to the social or conceptual relation. But what does this mean? Leibniz wrote: "I agree that there are degrees of accidental unity, that a regulated society has more unity than a confused mob and that an organized body or indeed a machine has more unity than a society. That is, it is more appropriate to conceive of them as a single thing because there is more relation between the component elements."[18] Relation, then, seems to be a function of interdependence. Elsewhere he wrote: "If the parts which act together for a common *purpose* more properly compose a substance than do those which are in contact, then all the parts of the India Company would much better constitute a real substance than would a pile of stones."[19] (Italics mine.) Interdependence and similarity of purpose relate entities and give them some degree of accidental unity. This theoretical scheme, that solidarity is a function of power (which we shall substitute for interdependence) and similarity, is of course repeated in all the sociological classics that deal with the subject.

Durkheim, Freud, and Toennies at approximately the same time established what is still our framework for the analysis of human relationships, but which adds little to Leibniz. Durkheim discussed similarity and functional dependence.[20] Freud discussed two bases for love: (1) narcissistic: when the other person resembles us as we are or were, or would like to be; and (2) functional: when the other person gives us tenderness or protection.[21] Finally Toennies distinguished: (1) friendship: "The simplest fellowship type is represented by a pair who live together in a brotherly, comradely, and friendly manner, and it is most likely to exist when those involved are of the *same* age, sex and sentiment or engaged in the *same* activity or have the *same* intentions, or when they are united by one idea" (emphasis mine), and (2) the authoritative type, such as the relation between a father and

[18] *Leibniz: Discourse on Metaphysics* 196.

[19] *Ibid.*, footnote on p. xiv.

[20] Emile Durkheim, *The Division of Labor in Society,* translated by George Simpson (Glencoe, Ill.: Free Press, 1933). The entire work develops the thesis that there are these two bases of solidarity.

[21] Sigmund Freud, "On Narcissism: An Introduction," in *Collected Papers,* vol. 4 (New York: Basic Books, 1959) 47.

son.[22] In short, relationship varies with similarity (to real and ideal self) and dependence or power.[23]

Less noted is Simmel's work which suggests a third basis: "All relations which people have to one another are based on their knowing something about one another. . . . One may say (without reservations which easily suggest themselves) that in all relations of a personally differentiated sort, intensity and nuance develop in the degree to which each party, by works and by mere existence, reveals itself to the other."[24]

Although emphasizing the significance of knowledge as a basis for classifying relationships, Simmel did not discuss the implication of this suggestion for the dualistic theories of relation popular at the time. In this paper we would like to stress the tripartite structure of social involvement: similarity, power, and knowledge.

The idea of the three bases makes sense, for each is a way of being another. If two people are similar they are, to a degree, the same. Likewise, if one person has power over another, the subordinate becomes the concrete embodiment of the purpose existing in the mind of the power-wielder; in a way, therefore, the slave is the master and vice versa. Finally, to the extent we know someone, that person exists in our minds, and we are the other. Similarity, power, and knowledge represent three ways of being another.

Finally, in a study of reactions to the death of President Kennedy, the extent of student reactions was found to be

[22] Ferdinand Toennies, *Community and Society,* translated by Charles Loomis (New York: Harper Torchbook, 1963) 252.

[23] Frederick summarized the historical discussion of the meaning of community as follows: "First, there is the debate as to whether community in the first instance simply exists, or whether it is willed. Secondly, there is the debate over whether the community, other values apart, is primarily a community of law or of love. Thirdly, there is the debate over whether community is organic or purposive." Carl Frederick, "The Concept of Community in the History of Political and Legal Philosophy" in Carl Frederick, ed., *Community* (New York: Liberal Arts Press, 1959) 23–24. "Willed," "law," and "purposive" refer to systems based on power; the other terms are more ambiguous but seem to imply the nonrational attraction that Toennies discussed, which occurs in groups connected via similarity and where the ethos is one of fundamental identity of the members of the group because of common blood.

[24] Kurt Wolff, *The Sociology of Georg Simmel* (Glencoe, Ill.: Free Press, 1950) 307.

related to these same three variables.[25] The variables worked differently for males and females, and the study leaves much to be desired, but it does offer some additional support for our tripartite theory of social involvement. This leads us to our third proposition: *The extent to which an aggregate is experienced as real depends upon the degree of similarity, power, and knowledge among its constituent parts.*

To summarize: The extent to which an aggregate is experienced as real depends upon: (1) the extent to which an aggregate has been solidified perceptually, (2) the degree of overlap between the perceptual and cognitive organizations, and (3) the degree of similarity, power, and knowledge among its constituent parts. One final comment: We should stress the significance of similarity, for it is involved in both the perceptual and cognitional levels of organization; thus an aggregate united by similarity will probably produce a greater sense of solidarity than one based on either power or knowledge.[26]

THE REWARDS OF FAMILY SOLIDARITY

Transcendence

The family is significant not only because it is so real, but also because it is the social institution most deeply rooted in the physical. Recently, the anthropologist Turner has stressed the transcendent quality of the physical:

> Among the earliest symbols produced by man are the three colours representing products of the human body, whose emission, spilling, or production is associated with a heightening of emotion—in other words, culture, the super-organic, has an intimate connection with the organic in its early stages, with the awareness of powerful physical experiences.

. . . .

[25] Joseph B. Tamney, "A Study of Involvement: Reactions to the Death of President Kennedy," unpublished manuscript. The entire paper concerns the relation between the assassination and the variables similarity, power, and knowledge.

[26] A fourth hypothesis should probably be added to our analysis: An aggregate is experienced as real to the extent that people say it is real. How far can the myth deviate from the "reality"?

The basic three [physical processes] are sacred because they have the power "to carry the man away," to overthrow his normal powers of resistance. Though immanent in his body they appear to transcend his consciousness.[27]

The physical transcends man, and thus attracts him. One of the sources of religious appeal is the inability of an individual to justify his own existence; every man finds a reason for living that lies outside his own uniqueness; every man seeks to transcend what he is, to justify his continuing to be. And the physical, because it is beyond our control and understanding (as of now), is experienced as a transcendent dimension of experience. Therefore, participation in it alleviates the need to justify our unique being.

Two obvious situations in which man experiences most clearly his participation in the physical are intercourse and birth, which two events are, of course, the foundation of the family—and thus the significance of this institution.

One of the attractions of the large family especially is that it allows the parents to be natural, that is to follow the dictates of their physiological processes, thus enhancing this sense of participation in the physical. The present widespread introduction of some degree of birth control will surely curtail, if not meaningfully eliminate, this sense of naturalness that has characterized family life in the past. The apparently inevitable introduction of control into sexual behavior would seem, therefore, to effectively do away with one of the primary sources of satisfaction of family life: participation in a transcendent physical world.

Appeal of Babies

An interesting fact is that people love babies, that is, not so much children as babies. One husband described his wife's behavior: "Occasionally we see a little baby and she wants to have another one. The other night we went over to some friends and she picked up their baby, a real cute little red-

27 Victor W. Turner, "Colour Classification in Ndembu Ritual" in Michael Banton, ed., *Anthropological Approaches to the Study of Religion* (New York: Praeger, 1966) 80, 82.

headed baby, and was playing with it when I came in the room. She said, 'You'd better get me out of here!' I feel the same way sometimes when I see a cute baby on TV or in a magazine."[28] This certainly is not an unusual event. Many people find it hard to resist babies. Why?

We suggest that the significance of the adult-baby relationship is that in it man comes close to experiencing a participation in a transcendent, presocialized world and that this is possible because the relationship is so contrary to Parson's and Shil's paradigm for a "solidarity interactive relationship."

> The polarity of gratification and deprivation is crucial here. An appropriate reaction on alter's part is a gratifying one to ego. If ego conforms with the norm, this gratification is in one aspect a reward for his conformity with it; the converse holds for the case of deprivation and deviance. The reactions of alter toward ego's conformity with or deviance from the normative pattern thus become sanctions to ego. Ego's expectations vis-à-vis alter are expectations concerning the roles of ego and of alter; and sanctions reinforce ego's motivation to conform with these role-expectations. Thus the complementarity of expectations brings with it the reciprocal reinforcement of ego's and alter's motivation to conformity with the normative pattern which defines their expectations.[29]

Parents, of course, feel involved with their babies; there is the blood relationship and the living together (and therefore spatial unity); perhaps there is a physical similarity, and certainly there is considerable power exercised by the parents. But all of these things can be said of children generally. What seems to distinguish our relation with babies is the comparative absence of expectations and norms—those things which Parsons and Shils believe essential to a solidary relationship. Our relation to a baby is precious because society, in the form of expectation, is absent from it.

Playing with children tends to be spontaneous. We react to the moment, not playing a pre-established role but letting ourselves go in response to the immediate situation. At such

[28] Rainwater, *op. cit.* 163.
[29] Talcott Parsons and Edward A. Shils, eds., *Toward a General Theory of Action* (Cambridge: Harvard University Press, 1952) 106.

times we feel real because: (1) We are responding to the immediate situation and thus have no sense of being a vehicle for the past. A spontaneous situation is a timeless event; we, the ones responsible for our acts, are identical with those carrying out the acts. Compare this spontaneous play with a man plagued by guilt, whose actions are repeatedly atonements for a past misdeed. Such a man feels that he is, and yet is not, responsible for his present penance. Only spontaneous behavior destroys the past and gives us the sense that our actions are fully ours. And (2) spontaneous acts are our acts, and do not belong to all those who have contributed to the description of some role, such as bank teller. In spontaneous play we are being ourselves in the fullest human sense; the absence of society in the sense of the absence of goals allows us to be real.[30]

In the previous section we discussed the conditions for experiencing a social aggregate as real. We now add that for an individual to experience himself fully as part of this aggregate, he must see purely himself in his behavior, which condition is most closely attained in spontaneous play. Playing with one's own children would be a situation, therefore, of very high solidarity.

But there is another reason for the importance of the comparative absence of society in such play, namely the absence of language. Many scholars have noted the strong sense of solidarity at a time of disaster. One student whom we interviewed soon after the assassination of President Kennedy made the following remark: "I felt deeply united with everybody, on the streets, on the campus, at the radio station. . . . Everybody's mind was occupied by one thought and this fact accounted for making millions of people one whole. It was so much so that no words were needed for communication. At least for the first hour after the assassination, I didn't feel the need to talk. I don't suppose anybody did. The expres-

---

[30] There seems to be a lack of recognition that probably the most important function of the family is to be a functionless social unit. Home offers a time and place to do nothing legitimately; at the same time relationships are maintained on the perceptual level, that is, members of a family are perceived, and therefore experienced, as a social unit even though no social activity takes place. Relations in the home are maintained and require little maintenance.

sions of people everywhere could say more than a long conversation."

This respondent firmly believed there was no need for conversation because everyone felt the same. But my interviews with forty students and Barber's with eight different work groups[31] revealed that there was not a uniform reaction to the assassination. Yet it is true that people perceived great similarity of response. Why?

The answer centers on the preponderance of low-information communication following the assassination. This event had affected people deeply; it was an emotional situation; given a rather limited behavioral repertory for emotional expression this meant that people observed each other behaving similarly. Moreover, the accompanying verbal communication transmitted little more information than these physiological symptoms. One student had to call her parents —"I just had to be reassured that they were feeling the way I did. I knew they were, but I had to be sure."

Following is a description of the telephone conversation:

Well, I got on and my mother said "hi" and I said "hi." And she said, "What can I say?" and I said, "Nothing, I just can't believe it." And then there was silence. Then my mother spoke with my father, and she said, "She's on the phone." And then my mother said, "I've been glued to the TV set," and I said, "So have I." And then my father got on the phone and said, "What can I say? I may not have agreed with him in all cases, but I admired him." And then I just said, "I thought he was a wonderful man; this is horrible." And then he said, "Did you call your sister, the one in Milwaukee?" and I said yes and that I was the one that told her. And then he said, "She didn't know about it?" and I said no and I said, "Don't forget to put the flag out." And then my mother got back on and she told me about my sister in Boston, because Boston is so familiar with the Kennedys. And then that's all, and she said, "All we can do is pray." That's all then, and I hung up. There wasn't very much we could say.

[31] James D. Barber, "Peer Group Discussion and Recovery from the Kennedy Assassination" in Bradley Greenberg and Edwin B. Parker, eds., *The Kennedy Assassination and the American Public* (Palo Alto: Stanford University Press, 1965) 118.

This conversation illustrates the low-information conversation that I believe characterized the nation after the assassination. Even though the communication is verbal, it is close to nonhuman forms of communication. One respondent wanted to talk, "Get it out of your system, curse a little bit, yell, scream, tell what we'd like to do to Oswald. . . . " The similar physiological symptoms and the predominance of nondiscriminatory verbal communication allowed sufficient communication to activate projective responses but not enough to disconfirm these projections.

Similar to a disaster, the near-absence of society in the form of language eliminates a source of divisiveness in the adult-baby relationship; it allows a maximum of projections and thus contributes to an unusual sense of high solidarity.

In short, playing with babies is probably the most common activity, lasting for any significant length of time,[32] which yields a very high sense of being part of a solidified world. This activity can yield such a result because of the absence of society in the twofold sense of the absence of goals and the absence of language. Further, we suggest that such experiences are rewarding because they relieve the individual of the sense of jutting out and, therefore, of the need to justify himself. Man becomes immersed and thus ceases to experience the problem of why he exists. Moreover, babies are extensions of our bodies, so that by relating to them we are, in a way, involving ourselves in the transcendent physical. Union with those precivilized creatures gives, then, not only high solidarity, but a sense of participation in the transcendent universe.[33]

At times adults play with each other as they play with babies, but these occasions are, I suspect, infrequent. There is at present no substitute for the adult-baby relationship, and until one is devised the reward of such a relationship will play a significant role in motivating childbirth. Especially in a society which has minimized the hardships of child rear-

[32] Sex of course provides heightened solidarity, but only for bursts of time.
[33] This sense of encountering a transcendent reality is heightened by very young children's ability to help us rediscover the world. They unmask it for us. Seeing it without our values and language, they help to free us from our cultural cocoon. Through them we encounter the "eternal."

ing, the continued presence of a baby in a home would seem desirable. From the perspective of solidarity, therefore, the attractiveness of the adult-baby relationship would seem likely to exert constant pressure toward high fertility rates.

Rewards of Adult Children

There seem to be two major rewards from grown children. One is self-extension:

> Workers may also attempt to cushion the impact of failure and to maintain an identification with the tradition of opportunity by projecting their unfulfilled ambitions upon their children—their extended ego, as it were. . . . ambition for a child may substitute for ambition for oneself.[34]
>
> The significance of these aspirations for children as a possible substitute for personal achievement emerged in the comment of a thirty-two-year-old machine operator who had taken his first job in the depths of the Great Depression: "I never had a chance, but I want my kids to go to college and do something better than factory work." The direct relationship which may exist between the hopes men have for their children and their own unfulfilled interests and desires is suggested by a worker who, having once played an instrument in a high school band, hoped that his son might become a professional musician, and by the would-be cartoonist who hoped that his four-year-old son would become an artist—seeing in his childish scribblings signs of some artistic capacity and interest.[35]

Failure breeds this desire for extension, but we must remember that death is a form of failure, and not attribute this motive only to the economically deprived.

The second reward is self-expansion; a mother remarked, "My oldest son is thoughtful and studious, the young one is a natural-born mechanic. I think that is what is interesting about a family; it's the variety you get in personalities and dispositions."[36] Having a large family is one way, perhaps the

[34] Ely Chinoy, *Automobile Workers and the American Dream* (Garden City, N.Y.: Doubleday, 1955) 126.
[35] *Ibid.* 127.
[36] Rainwater, *op. cit.* 165.

best way, of getting to know intimately a variety of people, thus broadening one's understanding of the world.

Grown children, then, offer self-extension and self-expansion.

Self-Extension: It is our contention that this reward will continually decline as a motive for fertility. Perhaps the most important reason for this concerns the change taking place in what is being extended. A study of India concluded that, "The most significant reason for desiring more children was found to be 'the need to ensure family survival!' "[37] In the past, and in some places today, children were needed to continue the family line; what was being extended was the family and not the individual mother or father. In modern, industrialized societies the extended family has become less real, so that the individuals who are a part of it can no longer experience their own survival in the continuance of the family name. It is no longer sufficient that a name and a history survive. For self-extension to be significant this mother and this father must gain a sense of continuance from the existence of this child.

The offspring, then, must be coded with the same blueprint that guides the parents, and this coding must be done by the parents. It is not sufficient that we meet people like us. Rather, to gain a sense of self-extension these individuals must be similar because we have willed them thus; these extensions must be willed into being as we will ourselves into existing. Self-extension requires, at least ideally, the continuance of the will.

To ensure this, parents must have sufficient power over their children so that they might form these offspring in their own image. However, increasing modernization means the continuous lessening of such control. In the process of removing the hardships associated with child rearing through increased child care facilities, we are removing power from the parents. To the degree we are successful in making child rearing pleasant, to the same degree we are eliminating the

---

[37] C. Chandrasekaran, "Recent Trends in Family Planning Research in India" in Berelson *et al., op. cit.* 553.

basis for self-extension as a fertility motive.[38]

Changes in the identity of the parents are also making self-extension harder to achieve. When a parent becomes involved in his work, it is difficult to look upon a child as his or her extension. To do so the child would have to be like the parent not only in mannerisms, skills, and personality but in career as well, and given the fact that occupational pursuits are more and more determined impersonally, outside the home, such similarity will probably decline from what it has been in close homes where parents were not involved in their work.

It follows, therefore, that if we can expect adults to become more involved in their careers, then a sense of self-extension would be less likely to occur. But such an expectation seems well-founded. Victor Fuchs has discussed the very significant fact that in the past decade we became the first "service economy," that is, the first nation in which more than half of the employed population was not involved in the production of food, clothing, houses, automobiles or other tangible goods.[39]

> For many decades, we have been hearing that industrialization has "alienated" the worker from his work, that the individual has no contact with the final fruit of his labor, and that the transfer from a craft society to one of mass production has resulted in depersonalization and in the loss of ancient skills and virtues.
>
> Whatever validity such statements may have had in the past, a question rises whether they now accord with reality. For the advent of a service economy implies a reversal of these trends. Employees in many service industries are clearly related to their work and often render a highly personalized service, of a kind that offers ample scope for the development and exercise of personal skills.[40]

[38] Moreover, the increasing independence of husband and wife means that each child will represent some sort of compromise between these two socializers and, therefore, satisfactorily represent neither. Just this occurrence, in fact, will lessen the parents' opposition to the loss of power because of some form of collective child rearing.

[39] Victor Fuchs, "The First Service Economy," *The Public Interest* 1, no. 2 (Winter 1966) 7.

[40] *Ibid.* 13.

Although automation will no doubt reach the service sector of our economy, it also seems certain that in the future work will be vastly different from the assembly line; specifically, it would seem to stress creativity, which requires both independence and spontaneity. If we compare the man on the assembly line who, while attaching his bolts to the machine-carcass, dreams of a wild affair with a movie star to a scientist concentrating on creating a human being, we see the difference between the past and the future. The adults of tomorrow will more fully be their work, will be more involved in their work in the same way that adults become involved in playing with babies. They will be their work, which means that self-extension will be increasingly difficult to experience.[41]

We assume, therefore, that self-perpetuation through fertility will become less and less meaningful: (1) because parents are losing control over their children, and (2) because adults are becoming more involved in their work, making meaningful parent-child similarity less likely.[42]

Self-Expansion: Whereas extension seems related to power and secondarily similarity, expansion appears to be related to knowledge. We enlarge ourselves by becoming others via understanding them. It seems quite possible that this reward will increase in significance because of the decline in power among the members of a family.

There is some evidence to support the hypothesis that self-revelation is inversely related to the amount of power in a relationship. Michelon has noted that honesty is one of the

[41] And, of course, the fact that women are working more and more means that this argument applies to both sexes.

[42] Westoff has written: "There is neither evidence to support the hypothesis that job or career interests stand opposed to familial interests or . . . that there exists a direct relationship between extrafamilial participation and interest in and liking for children." Charles F. Westoff *et al., Family Growth in Metropolitan America* (Princeton, N.J.: Princeton University Press, 1961) 304. What must be studied is the relation between involvement at work and involvement at home, and the relation between involvement and interest, by which we mean attention or the focusing of energy; since interest refers to energy it is, unlike involvement, a scarce commodity. It seems to us that involvement in work would lessen the expenditure of interest in the home, because of the loss of the self-extension reward, thus lessening involvement in the home.

privileges of retirement: "For the first time the individual is truly independent. He can say what he pleases."[43] Similarly, Moustakis quotes a leper to the effect that in the colony there is an openness;[44] it is rather difficult to assert control over a dying man. Finally, Levenson's report of a study carried out in a utility company noted that, "When things are going well, where both employees and company accept their dependence on each other, people are reluctant to express openly whatever feelings of hostility may arise toward important figures in authority."[45] Power seems to inhibit communication.

If we are right in predicting a continued decline in power within the family, it seems quite possible that self-expansion will become an increasingly important motive for fertility. Would such a motive lead to unlimited childbearing?

We suggest that the conscious pursuit of self-expansion will lead to family limitation. Aristotle thought somewhat similarly: "One cannot be a friend to many people in the sense of having friendship of the perfect type with them, just as one cannot be in love with many people at once. . . . it is not easy for many people at the same time to please the same person very greatly, or perhaps even to be good in his eyes. One must, too, acquire some experience of the other person and become familiar with him, and that is very hard."[46] Understanding requires time and effort or interest, which is a scarce resource. As family size increases, interest must be dissipated and understanding per person decline. It seems, therefore, that the motive of self-expansion contains a built-in brake.

It seems relatively clear why adults might seek self-expansion through children. Birth allows us all to be little gods; it takes the guessing out of self-expansion. Why gamble on making and retaining friends when one can be sure of having

43 L. C. Michelson, "The New Leisure Class," *American Journal of Sociology* 59, no. 4 (January 1954) 343.

44 Clark Edward Moustakis, *Loneliness* (Englewood Cliffs, N.J.: Prentice-Hall, 1961) 97.

45 Harry Levenson, *Men, Management and Mental Health* (Cambridge: Harvard University Press, 1962) 94.

46 McKeon, *op. cit.* 479.

offspring? The method of having children would seem to take the insecurity out of personal growth through understanding others.

But there seems to be a basis for questioning whether children will appreciate this. Aristotle wrote: "This is why it would not seem open to a man to disown his father (though a father may disown his son); being in debt, he should repay, but there is nothing by doing which a son will have done the equivalent of what he has received, so that he is always in debt."[47] Hobbs believed that when one friend did something for another that the latter could never match, the friendship was over, for no one likes to be continually reminded of his inability to repay another. Given the decline in parental power that has already begun, will children prefer parents to peers, if associating with the former always means being reminded of their debt?

As we enter an age of control, birth will be an unmatchable gift from a parent to a child. Will people communicate as freely and as deeply within a debtors prison as they do in the freedom of pure friendship? If the purpose of communication is to connect and unify self and environment, the answer would seem to be no, for the matchless parental gift would forever prevent a child from feeling one with his parent; first he would always be a debtor. We suggest, therefore, that possibly children will decline to play their part and will refuse to be the vehicle of parental self-expansion.

Unfortunately, however, we have hardly begun to answer the questions related to the significance and extent of understanding within a family. Somewhere Yeats wrote that "the intellect of man is forced to choose perfection of the life or of the work." Certainly interest is scarce, and an adult who likes his work will expend more energy on it than someone who does not. What then will be the effect of technological changes, which will involve future adults in their work to a greater extent, on the amount of interest available for the home world? What is the relation between interest and knowledge? Is there a critical amount of interest necessary for some understanding, after which little amounts of inter-

---

[47] *Ibid.* 494.

est have high payoffs? Is it true the more we really come to understand something, the more we realize how little we know about it? These and other questions must be answered if we are to predict the relation between self-expansion and fertility.

Although we have suggested, then, that personal growth might become an increasingly important motive for fertility in the future, we have also noted two problems: (1) Understanding would seem to be inversely related to family size, so that self-expansion would seem to be a self-braking motive for fertility. And (2) it is possible that children may not play the game, thus eliminating the motive.

CONCLUSION

The paper began by suggesting that the present conditions limiting fertility might cease to exist and raised the question whether in a time of affluence and child care facilities any fertility-limiting factors would exist. We restricted the discussion to viewing childbirth from the perspective of solidarity.

Our conclusions were: (1) fertility-control would eliminate the rewards of participation in a transcendent physical world; (2) in a world where child rearing involves little pain, babies would be especially appealing and be a spur to fertility; (3) declining parental power and increasing involvement in work will effectively eliminate self-perpetuation as a fertility reward; and (4) self-expansion will increase in importance but is self-braking and possibly might fail to become a significant motive of fertility because of a child's inability to be a friend to a parent. If this last reward does become significant it would limit the effect of the appeal of babies on fertility. But if it does not, would this leave fertility at the mercy of the attractiveness of infants? We doubt it. If parents are unable to anticipate any significant reward from their grown children, birth would lead to a painful life, for perceptual relations would continue with these children even in the absence of meaningful social relations. Thus having babies in a time when children and parents could not be friends would mean eventually suffering continued alienation. From the viewpoint of solidarity it would seem that if parents and children are not able to overcome the gift of birth, child rearing will be perceived as a potential source of pain, and adults will seek to develop a way of life that does not involve having children.

DISCUSSION

In separate discussions, John S. Dunne, C.S.C., and George Hagmaier, C.S.P., review Mr. Tamney's paper, "Family Solidarity and Fertility." Father Dunne considers the motivation at work in society and suggests that the lack of immediacy in life may be the shortcomings of our society and solutions. Father Hagmaier mentions some of the problems of community education as a means of teaching responsible parenthood. He questions the status of coercive education, suggesting that it may be necessary because of the inadequacy of other solutions.

DUNNE: I found Mr. Tamney's paper extremely interesting. It touched upon the basic motivations at work in a society, particularly that which I consider most fundamental: the endeavor to solve the problem of death.

Mr. Tamney suggests that self-perpetuation as a fertility reward will probably be eliminated by declining parental power and increasing involvement in work. In a society more primitive than our own this type of motivation would be much stronger. For instance, in a patriarchal society like the one found in the Bible in a story of Abraham, Isaac, and Jacob, self-perpetuation through one's offspring is the characteristic means of overcoming death. Abraham's hope is his posterity. He has no hope for a life after death, but he hopes to perpetuate himself through Isaac. Such hope is probably typical of nomadic and patriarchal societies. In societies still more primitive, hunting and food-gathering societies, there is usually no sense of a cumulative past. On the contrary, there is often a severing of relations with the dead after burial. There is no tradition in such societies, and so life tends to begin pretty much from scratch, the only significant time being the individual lifetime. Because of a lack of history and tradition such societies are very static. Only where there is a tradition accumulating with heroes and past history, it seems, can there be any sense of unique events and of new things happening in the present.

A modern society presents a strong contract with both of these types of society. The sense of history and of a cumulative past can be found in all the higher civilizations, ancient and modern, but it has been accentuated in modern societies with the appearance of movements which are historically oriented. The modern man, even the one who is not greatly educated, can be caught in these movements and have a sense of participation in history by which he can find a solution to the problem of death. By casting his lot with some historical movement, by making some cause his own project in life, he triumphs over death. The success of the cause is his success; its failure is his failure. Thus, the modern revolutionary hopes that he will be "vindicated by history," and the modern democratic statesman like Lincoln resolves, "that these dead shall not have died in vain." For if the cause is triumphant, then the man who dedicated his life to it is vindicated by history, but if it is lost, then such a man will have died in vain. The sense of history and of a cumulative past is characteristic of all the higher civilizations including the ancient ones, but the sense of participation in a historical movement is perhaps peculiar to the more modern.

The important thing in regard to fertility and childbearing is that if the problem of death is solved on the historic level, then the motivation for having children is lessened. If we were living in a more primitive society where the problem of death was solved by having children, then the whole structure of motives would be quite different. One of Mr. Tamney's main points, it seems, is that this motivation is decreasing in our society because of its very modernity and its sense of history.

His other points, however, seem antithetical. There is a human desire for immediate physical experience and for participation in the physical world. There is the human significance of intercourse and birth. These factors favor fertility and childbearing. The way they figure for the modern man would be something like this: When we live on this high historical level, participating in movements and historical events, we feel a lack in ourselves, a loss of substance, a loss of humanity. It is the lack of immediate relationships, the lack of touch with immediate physical reality. Modern society for this reason can be very unsatisfying. The modern solution to the problem of death on the high level of historical consciousness is an attraction away from childbearing and is a motive involving one in work and projects. The shortcomings of modern society and of its solutions to life's problems, on the other hand, may lead us to seek fulfillment in childbearing and in the immediacies of the family.

Both sides appear in Mr. Tamney's paper, but I would like to relate them in the following way. I think that in every society there is some kind of solution to the problem of death and, thus, to the problems of life. In the classical Greek and Roman republics, for example, there was the ideal of performing immortal deeds; in the later Roman empire there was the ideal for running the gamut of experience; in modern societies there is the ideal of appropriating one's life and one's times, involving oneself in the course of history. Such solutions embody, I believe, the most powerful motivations at work in societies, yet, there is usually some shortcoming in them which causes the societies ultimately to decline and fall. Perhaps, there is some such flaw in the modern type of solution, and perhaps it involves the lack of immediacy in a life lived on the historic plane. If so, we may have our finger on something which is destined to play an important role in the ultimate fate of our society.

HAGMAIER: I am not a sociologist or a philosopher and I thought both of these disciplines were uniquely represented in the paper. Some psychological insights especially intrigued me. I have decided to comment today as an educator-therapist, particularly as an educator who is interested in how one prepares the community for responsible parenthood. There is not much on this particular subject anywhere, and the more I consult with the few educators who are giving it some thought, the more confused I become.

I suspect the paradoxical nature of this paper was to some

extent deliberately intended by Mr. Tamney, particularly in the area of community education. I presume that in some way all educators for responsible parenthood would hope that there will be fewer babies born in the future. Who should have fewer babies, who should have a planned number, and who should have more are very tricky questions. The categories which the educator uses to arrive at answers are complex indeed. In some localities, because of population pressures, there should be fewer babies in terms of the entire social setting; in individual families limitation will be called because of the undesirable population explosion within one family as a result of too close spacing or too many children.

Our guidelines must come through continuing research. The papers we have heard so far, including Mr. Tamney's, suggest that we should stop haggling as to whether the sociologist or the psychologist should have the final say about methods and objectives. Rather there should be a very careful listening of each to the other, a collaborative reinforcement of the good insights both have to give.

Once the goals are clear, the questions still remain: "Can we really determine, ahead of time, methods of education which will work? Can we really program the future in this area?"

We face at once the word which has been getting headlines recently: coercion. There are concerned moralists, including the American bishops, who seem to feel that any effort toward educating for responsible parenthood carries with it the grave danger of violating personal freedom. The implication is sharpened by the urgency of the issue. Many behavioral scientists point with mounting alarm to a precariously burgeoning population, especially in certain impoverished pockets of the country and the world. "We haven't time to make long-range plans and undertake delicate approaches to public enlightenment." The high fertility rate, the large incidence of illegitimacy preclude any leisurely attempt to motivate many people to a highly personal regulation of birth. The implication is, of course, that a crash program of contraceptive propaganda will mislead or intimidate potential users and prevent truly responsible decisions on their own. The danger of coercion, therefore, seems a very real one.

This threat makes sense in terms of the many subtle unconscious factors which underlie the decision of parents to limit or not limit their families. Some of these intriguing paradoxes are touched upon by Mr. Tamney.

He mentions, for example, the symbolic importance of parents participating in the transcendental physical world at moments of intercourse and birth, and suggests that outside or "artificial" interference will produce a less satisfactory and imperfect experience. I suggest, however, that such a possibility must be balanced with the likelihood that too frequent births can also become, especially for the woman, an unpleasant, unsatisfactory, and damaging prospect. Anticipating the real possibility of conception, with all its resulting burdens, can also color the psychological quality of intercourse, impairing the desirable free and spontaneous character of the sexual encounter.

Another observation of Mr. Tamney's carries with it the likelihood of a dilemma. Granted that expanding child care facilities may remove many burdens from the shoulders of parents and encourage large families as a result. Still, the very perceptive suggestion that adults enjoy having babies around—that the little ones are nice to be with—carries with it some disturbing inferences.

Parents—especially mothers—can use their children for their own inadequately filled emotional needs, can become too absorbed in them, can prevent them from growing up, precisely because when they are young they make few demands and bring highly gratifying returns. With the passing of time, feelings of ambivalence develop and the immature parent, not able to deal adequately with these feelings, can communicate his or her anxiety to the child.

It was interesting for me, visiting the nursery schools in Russia and observing parents and children in the kibbutzim in Israel, to observe considerable uneasiness on the part of many mothers who had misgivings about leaving their children in the care of substitute parents a good part of the time. Some Israeli mothers, in particular, felt very guilty in not being able to tuck their youngsters in bed at night or not having them around more. They felt, somehow, that they were less "motherly" in acquiescing to the children's cottage system.

My point is that it may be too simple to suggest that more outside help will make for happier families. Anxious parents, doting on the agreeable presence of babies in the home, will still manipulate their children into a dependency relationship which may make it even more difficult for the child to pull away into adulthood and become the agreeable and liberated friend to the parent that Mr. Tamney hopes for.

When we take into account these and other possibly conflicting subconscious influences motivating individual parents, we face the difficulty of programming a single educational plan for the community in the area of responsible parenthood. I suspect that we will need as many approaches to individual families as we seem to need in meeting the quite different problems of various nationalities and sections within our country. I am rather pessimistic about the ease with which we can do this.

Individual psychological dynamics cannot be minimized. For example, complex emotional undercurrents are undoubtedly at work in the woman who consciously agrees to take the pill but who somehow forgets, often at the most inopportune time. We see similar behavior in certain alcoholics whose wives nag them to take a drug which will prevent their drinking. Somehow they forget, and once again the wife has a problem on her hands. Such forgetfulness can be an elaborate outlet for repressed hostility, a subtle way to get back at one's insensitive spouse— keeping an argument going by getting pregnant about it!

Father Bernard Häring's writings, if I understand them correctly, seem to be saying something very perceptive. Using somewhat traditional natural law concepts, Father Häring proposes that ultimately parents who have thoughtfully, prayerfully, and with counsel considered the various implications of future pregnancies, may be encouraged to practice that method of birth prevention which, *for them, least interferes* with the naturalness of the sexual act.

However, we face a challenge in adopting this pastoral approach which has not, until now, received adequate attention, chiefly because of the unprepared state of many Catholics toward self-directed problem-solving. Many parishioners, educated or not, are confused as they face dilemmas in their moral lives when they are told, "follow your conscience to the best of your ability"

97

—a dictum accepted in theory by our traditional theology, but little practiced. "I thought the Church is supposed to tell me what to do" is the response of many bewildered penitents, particularly those who have never before thought for themselves in any moral area.

There are undoubtedly some couples—perhaps quite a few—who would be perfectly content to follow this or that advice proposed by some authoritative voice in the Church, whatever that advice might be. But how is the priest or counselor able to determine beforehand if this particular person or couple is disposed to such easy acquiescence—or whether, instead, they may be enmeshed in all sorts of complex, unconscious doubts and anxieties hidden from the counselor and even unknown to themselves, which will not make it possible for them to be easily reassured.

PART THREE

The Microanalysis of the Family and Fertility

MARVIN B. SUSSMAN

5. FAMILY INTERACTION AND FERTILITY

In this paper I will pose some propositions and hypotheses
and suggest a number of personal and societal variables
related to fertility. Family interaction can be viewed from
a number of perspectives. One perspective accounts for interaction among members of a nuclear unit; another views interaction between family units such as those linked together
in an urban kinship network along generational or bilateral
lines; and still another considers interaction of the nuclear
unit or the kinship network with other societal systems, such
as welfare, religious, educational, and economic. In using
any one of these perspectives, fertility is the dependent variable and interaction is the independent one.

In studying interaction between family members of a nuclear unit, it is necessary to consider those variables which
can be described as personal or individual. The focus is upon
situations, events, and personal characteristics which affect
the decision-making process regarding having or not having
a child. Such personal variables are values, goals, education,
religion, socio-economic level, and capacity for interpersonal
relationships. The notion is that, given a set of conditions

outside the boundaries of the nuclear unit, a decision to have a child is based upon the interaction among participants within the system. The nature of this interaction is related to these personal variables and the specific postures assumed by each individual. One consequence of interaction is change in the individual's stance and behavior. The family is a dynamic interaction system, and changes in attitudes or behavior of any one member of the family affect those of every other one. The sum is greater than the parts because of the many intricate interpersonal and intrapersonal positive and negative relationships.

Outside the nuclear unit one finds a set of variables, which we may call societal, that appear to influence the decisions made within the nuclear unit. Each individual brings into the interaction postures and orientations which reflect these societal imperatives. During the past decade researchers, such as Freedman,[1] Kiser and Whelpton,[2] Hoffman and Wyatt,[3] Rainwater,[4] Goldberg,[5] Westoff,[6] Hill, Stycos, and Back,[7] have proposed that changes in the roles of women and consequently those of men are a result of technological advances

[1] R. Freedman, "Fecundity and Family Planning in the White Population of the United States: 1955," in *Thirty Years of Research in Human Fertility* (New York: Milbank Memorial Fund, 1959) 61–73; *Family Planning, Sterility, and Population Growth,* with P. K. Whelpton and A. A. Campbell (New York: McGraw-Hill, 1959); "American Studies of Family Planning: A Review of Major Trends and Issues," in Clyde V. Kiser, ed., *Research in Family Planning* (Princeton, N.J.: Princeton University Press, 1962) 211–27.

[2] P. K. Whelpton and Clyde V. Kiser, "Fertility Planning and Fertility Rates by Socio-economic Status," in P. K. Whelpton and Clyde V. Kiser, eds., *Social and Psychological Factors Affecting Fertility* (New York: Milbank Memorial Fund, 1950) 2, 359–416; Clyde V. Kiser, "The Indianapolis Study of Social and Psychological Factors Affecting Fertility," in Clyde V. Kiser, ed., *Research in Family Planning* (Princeton, N.J.: Princeton University Press, 1962) 149–66.

[3] L. W. Hoffman and F. Wyatt, "Social Change and Motivations for Having Larger Families: Some Theoretical Considerations," *Merrill-Palmer Quarterly* 6, 235–44.

[4] L. Rainwater, *Family Design: Marital Sexuality, Family Size, and Contraception* (Chicago: Aldine, 1965).

[5] D. Goldberg, "The Fertility of Two Generation Urbanites," *Population Studies* 12, no. 3, 214–22; "Another Look at the Indianapolis Fertility Data," *Milbank Memorial Fund Quarterly* 38, no. 1 (1960) 23–26.

[6] C. Westoff, *Family Growth in Metropolitan America* (Princeton, N.J.: Princeton University Press, 1961).

[7] R. Hill, J. M. Stycos, and K. Back, *The Family and Population Control* (Chapel Hill: University of North Carolina Press, 1959).

in our society, the increase, in maternal employment, the growing attractiveness of the mother role, the rise in loneliness and alienation in modern urban society and, conversely, the larger opportunity system for many in the urban society, the increasing pervasiveness of religious attitudes, the rise of educational levels, and changing economic conditions; these are significant variables affecting decision-making in regard to fertility and other matters.

It may be that I have assigned too powerful an influence and independence to societal variables and that, while they affect intrafamily transactions, their effects are mitigated by the form and character of the interaction. Societal variables stand potentially as independent ones with interaction as a "screening" determinant of whether societal variables will be activated and influential in the interactional context.

Researchers like Lee Rainwater, Lois Hoffman, and Frederick Wyatt have concentrated their work largely on explaining the relationship of societal variables to human fertility. One should not overlook the demographic approach used by such investigators as Duncan, Bogue, Kiser, Whelpton, and others. There are, of course, psychoanalytic explanations as well as those derived from psychology, where major work has been done on motivation to have children. There is some beginning work on the processes and mechanisms of interaction in relation to decision making. Strodtbeck is attempting to ascertain and predict the cognitive processes by which AFDC mothers make decisions. In the data uncovered by Rainwater and Mirra Komarovsky, decisions about family size are usually adhered to when mutually arrived at by parents in open communication with each other.

In spite of all of these researches and efforts at explanation, much of what we know is derived from inferences about the importance of societal factors. Take the issue of technological advances which have produced less labor in the home and, therefore, have made available more leisure time for the woman to pursue other interests. She can seek gainful employment in the occupational world or take on new roles which enable her to give creative expression to her abilities and, therefore, be a better mate to her husband and a better mother to her children. The availability of leisure time and

103

the technological revolution in the home would mean, for some women, the need to have fewer children. For others it might be an incentive to have a "large" family, because creative expression can be attained through childbearing and rearing roles and there is safety in the knowledge that one is fulfilling societal expectations by staying at home and taking care of one's children.

Further analysis of this issue requires accounting for the religious identification of the individual, personality, and other cultural variables. The issue is by no means clear, and our level of knowledge is limited by inferential analysis about the personal considerations and dynamics involved in the decision to control or not control fertility. It is likely that our knowledge is scarce because of the difficulties—methodological and ethical—in getting at what people really think and actually do concerning human reproduction. The best we do is to find what people say and think they want regarding the number of children; then, through follow-up studies, discover the actual number they have; and then demonstrate the differences between stated desire and actual number, according to class and ethnic backgrounds and other variables. We do know some of the circumstances, reasons, and feelings of individuals in using or not using contraceptive devices.

Donald Bogue concludes from his research and that of others such as Westoff, Freedman, etc., that the great majority of the working class, middle and upper class (except strict Catholics) who are ineffective users of contraceptives (only about 10 per cent of this population) are neurotics who are impulse-ridden in many sectors of their lives. Aside from the lower-lower class, most Americans have the number of children they want. The lower-lower class are affected by ignorance, rural backgrounds, apathy and fatalism, fear, and factors of marital conflict. Rainwater and Komarovsky conclude that intercourse-connected contraceptives are not used—or used poorly—by couples who have segregated role relationships, who fail to communicate, and couples in which the individuals feel alienated from each other. These conditions are much more likely to occur in the lower-lower class and especially among Negroes.

These conditions and processes do not explain the more

dynamic and idiosyncratic factors in making a decision contrary to expectations. Does the condition of real or perceived crisis or euphoria produce deviant (unexpected) behavior regarding fertility? Why is it that a couple who have employed a contraceptive device for a reasonable period of time will suddenly stop using it without any logical explanation and will virtually abandon a family planning program? We just do not know what occurs in the inner room of the family and have only slight knowledge of what occurs on the marital bed.

One major proposition in a study of personal factors affecting decision making in fertility is to consider sex relations as crisis resolution. I make this statement realizing fully its negative cast and that the desire to have a child grows out of mutuality, common values, and the desire to express warmth and to give joy. But I am trying to explain the failure to follow a prescribed regimen and the nonlogical and nonrational factors in fertility decision making.

Starting with this proposition of crisis resolution, one could add that in serious crises and problems there enters the element of human reproduction along with sexual intercourse. Our almost total disregard, ambivalence toward, and denial of human sexuality have resulted in our ignoring the therapeutic consequences of sexual intercourse in resolving marital conflicts and in providing security, identification, and solidarity to individuals when threatened from the outside. Under extreme threat and conditions which appear to have finality and which are uncontrollable by the individuals, the added dimension of abandonment of established procedures occurs. The urge to create becomes basic; it is as if man has returned to the primordial instincts so fundamental to the continuity of the human species. It is characteristic that after families have experienced the loss of a child they begin, almost immediately, efforts to conceive another. On a societal level we notice rises in the birth rate immediately after crises; the phenomenon of increased birth rate during wartime finds logic in this explanation. While this remains undocumented, marriage counselors consistently report that clients who are seeking help to prevent a divorce but are on the verge of obtaining one resort to having a child in an effort to save the marriage through pregnancy. What is unreported is whether this is a mutual effort or one by a single partner attempting to maintain the marriage.

If the proposition is reasonable and one accepts the further notion that family interaction is based upon a pattern of unequal reciprocity whereby individuals are contending for particular advantage within the reciprocal relationship, then one concludes that conflict and contention are ever present in marital interaction and that sex relations become an important technique for handling the consequences of conflict. On a purely statistical basis, one could expect the incidence of conception to be greater among individuals who have increased sexual intercourse, whether a contraceptive device is used or not. In other words, the more frequent the intercourse, the greater the opportunity to have an accident. If one adds to this the notion of crisis—either societal or personal—whereby individuals can not control their creative urges, he has one possible insight into the dynamics and, to some degree, the mechanisms employed in decision making regarding fertility.

In stating such propositions there is always the danger of being accused of denying or relegating to obscurity the obvious: couples have another child out of love for and joy in each other; conflict and crisis may result in sterility rather than fertility; sex relations can be more enjoyable to both husbands and wives when there is a close, mutual relationship; and wives particularly are disinterested—or actively dislike—sex when roles are segregated and there is little communication. According to Rainwater and Komarovsky, sex is viewed by the majority of husbands and wives as (a) a tension reliever and (b) a positive force for a sense of intimacy and mutuality. I recognize these alternatives and their possibilities in providing partial explanations for a segment of the population; yet I hold to other likely expositions.

A second and related observation is that the processes and mechanisms of communication among marital pairs vary extensively and that some utilize a rationalistic model of communication while others rely heavily on the nonverbal, a symbolic interaction model. Some individuals communicate and interact with others more in terms of feelings (visceral response) than on a scientific, logical, and rational basis. This does not mean that rationality and logic do not enter into their decisions. Individuals characterized as visceral respondents may understand the rationale of planning a family but enjoy too much the illogic of their actions, their responses to moods, feelings, and the problems posed by their irrational behavior, so that their lives take on meaning by nonconformity. Couples who are more verbal, more systematic, more rational, and scientific are much more guided by norms and rules and are much more establishment-oriented. Again, this is an observation which might provide the bases for a research project examining the quality and character of marital communication and its relationship to fertility. I should say at this point that Clark Vincent[8] has made a distinctive contribution to our thinking in suggesting to family sociologists that they conceptualize problems of family interaction—namely, interaction between parents and children—somewhat differently from those between marital partners. As he suggests, the problems, issues, and companionate methodologies are related but different.

It is now appropriate to consider the power and influence of societal factors in affecting fertility by taking a serious look at the kinship network in urban society and to examine whether being in a viable kin network of nuclear-related families and engaging in meaningful interaction involving reciprocal patterns of exchange of services, aid, and social activities have any important relationship to fertility. In another paper I have posited the bases upon which a viable nuclear-related kinship network exists in urban society; these bases are rooted in exchange of unequal reciprocities which in time become institutionalized in the form of expectations.[9]

[8] Clark Vincent, "Mental Health and the Family," *Journal of Marriage and the Family* 29, no. 1 (February 1967) 18–39.

[9] Marvin B. Sussman, "Theoretical Bases for an Urban Kinship Network System," paper read at the annual meeting of the National Council on Family Relations, October, 1966, Minneapolis, Minnesota. For a review of the kinship network notion, see "Kin Family Network: Unheralded Structure in Current Conceptualizations of Family Functioning," with L. Burchinal, *Marriage and Family Living* 24 (1962) 231–40. "The Urban Kin Network in the Formulation of Family Theory," The Ninth International Seminar on Family Research, Tokyo, Japan, 1965, forthcoming in Rene Koenig, ed., *Yearbook of International Sociological Associations*.

One could study the predisposing factors affecting the personal decision-making process by examining the availability of resources to marital couples of childbearing age. To what extent are they within kinship networks which have exchange mechanisms, service troops, financial resources, and emotional support? The work to date on kinship relations suggests that the intergenerational linkage is perhaps the most viable and forms the backbone of the urban kin network. How established are the expectations of grandparents, among different class and cultural groups, concerning the bearing and number of children? To what extent do they provide the emotional, service, and financial support for their young married children?

In treating intergenerational and kinship activity in fertility, one should also consider economic and value factors. Rainwater finds that most parents, on all income levels, think it is right and good to have large families, with the only deterrent being an economic one for each family. Only among the highly educated does one find the value that the wife should have time and energy for her fulfillment as a person aside from being a wife and mother. It is this group, too, that values small families because this frees the husband and wife for a close interpersonal relationship.

In this discussion we have assumed the continuity of relationships between nuclear family units along generational and bilateral kin lines. The other side of the coin is characterized by discontinuity, and the question can be raised as to how parental interference may affect the decision to have a child and the number of children. We now have enough publicized cases to indicate that, in order to legitimatize an elopement and forestall the obtaining of an annulment or parental pressures to effect a separation or divorce, a widespread practice among young couples is for the girl to become pregnant. These couples handle generational relationships by pregnancy. Another component of the pregnant bride phenomenon is the potentiality of effective manipulation of parents by the young couple, especially among middle-class families, when both sets of parents are eager to have their children college-educated. The parents most often continue to finance the married couple through college, while the young husband or wife uses the spouse as a buffer against the strings and demands of the parents providing the money. This pattern frequently has been interpreted as the pregnant bride's display of neurotic symptoms. In most instances it can more accurately be interpreted as the young couple's response to parental and societal denial of adult status to young people until they have completed their formal education, are well placed in an occupation, and have had their first child. It is more indicative of the ambiguity over the lines of the life-cycle stages—those between adolescence and adulthood—than neurotic symptoms.

One test of the influence of the family kinship network would be a study comparing family networks as to their attitudes and experiences concerning fertility. If the network has influence in developing the stance concerning fertility of its members, one would expect that, in all nuclear units of childbearing age within a viable network, the family size would differ very little. The expectation would be that the network had internalized values of smallness or bigness and that particular units were influenced by their membership within the kin network. The network in this instance provides the ethos for a policy and practice concerning fertility and utilizes its voluntary organizational apparatus to enable each individual unit to obtain its desired objective. This notion stems from research done in other areas, such as that of maternal employment.[10] One finds, for example, that in some communities, where the practice of the mother being employed outside the home is acceptable, working mothers appear to make good adjustment to both their outside jobs and to their role in the home, and there is an increased incidence of mothers gainfully employed. In communities where maternal employment is viewed negatively, the woman is usually under stress concerning her marital roles and makes a poorer adjustment on her job. Without community support

[10] Ruth E. Hartley, "What Aspects of Child Behavior Should be Studied in Relation to Maternal Employment," ·Research Issues Related to the Effects of Maternal Employment on Children (New York: Social Science Research Center, The Pennsylvania State University, June, 1966) 41–50; Marvin B. Sussman, "Needed Research on the Employed Mother," Marriage and Family Living 23 (1961) 368–73.

she strongly feels loneliness and alienation.

In summary, family interaction can be approached from several perspectives: (1) among members of a nuclear unit, (2) between family units, and (3) between the nuclear unit or the kinship network and other societal systems. In considering fertility and family interaction, fertility is the dependent variable and interaction the independent variable. These independent variables may be personal (sentiment, feeling, sexuality, intelligence, and so forth) or they may be societal (technological advances, maternal employment, the role of the mother, characteristics of modern urban society, religious attitudes, economic conditions, etc.), and both types of variables should be considered in discussing family interaction and fertility.

The propositions posed in this paper are that: (1) sex relations are used as a means of crisis resolution and are an important factor in decision making regarding fertility, (2) the processes and mechanisms of communication between marital partners are related to fertility, and (3) a number of societal factors have a screening effect upon interaction and subsequently affect decisions regarding fertility. Many of these factors have been studied for their relationship to fertility.[11] A potentially fruitful field of investigation is the activities of the kin network in modern society regarding support or nonsupport of the childbearing behavior of its members. The kin network is an extension of the primary group, and its influence has been ignored because of our preoccupation with a theoretical stance which relegates the family to a minor position in the modern age of complex organizations. It is my contention that the societal factor of the kin network may be the most important of all those indicated as affecting fertility.

The need for more research on the dynamics and mechanisms of interaction regarding fertility is obvious, and this research will require inventive minds and creative methodology. The examination of the role of the kin group in

[11] Catherine Chilman has an excellent review of population dynamics and poverty in the United States and its implications for family planning. She covers some of the major findings on societal factors affecting fertility decisions. *Growing Up Poor* (Washington, D.C.: U.S. Government Printing Office, 1966).

fertility behavior requires initially a theoretical posture embracing awareness of its existence and the functions it performs in the lives of family members. Then are required determination of the network in a given community and surveys and longitudinal studies of its utilization in fertility behavior, especially the role of kin members as socialization agents. Research is needed also as to the impact of family size and child spacing on (a) marital stability and satisfaction, (b) development of children, and (c) escape from poverty.

Finally we need more conclusive studies on the relationship of values about the kind of marriage one wants and the kind of relationship one wants with his children to desired family size and contraceptive effectiveness. The more one stresses individuality, psychological intimacy, mutuality of relationships, democratic family life, is it more likely that fertility will be carefully controlled by mutual husband-wife decision making? This is the most widely held position today.

FRED L. STRODTBECK
PAUL G. CREELAN

6. THE INTERACTION LINKAGE BETWEEN FAMILY SIZE AND SEX-ROLE IDENTITY*

In this paper we offer a comment upon the interaction opportunity system as it elaborates itself when a progressively larger number of siblings turn to the same parent for guidance and love.

The first third of the paper is devoted to the familiar topic of family size and intelligence. With this discussion we introduce a paradigm in terms of which one asks: What are the conditions under which it may be said that family size has an effect on a given characteristic? Then, and this is more important, one must ask: What is the nature of the family in order for the effect attributable to size have arisen? One considers what is associated with a given difference, then what is the nature of a system such that it would be changed by size in this manner.

Our intention in juxtaposing intelligence with sex-role identity, then relating both to family size, is not just to

* The authors wish to express their appreciation to William E. Bezdek and Donald Goldhamer for their assistance and kindness in permitting the use in this article of passing reference to materials which they are in the process of preparing for publication.

113

create a heuristic device to bring before this audience a well-worked classroom example. The state of our knowledge is much more tentative. At a time when the management of family size is receiving so much attention, one becomes curious about—and this is a favorite phrase—the unanticipated social consequences of modification in family size. While one may agree that our knowledge is not now adequate to the task, it is viewed as important that we are learning to ask better questions. By treating two examples—one well worked out, the other quite speculative—we attempt to set a more general question of the strategy for the next step. Of the many questions which might be asked, what are the questions which would help us to create a model of the interdependence between personality and society modified by a structural consideration such as family size?

FAMILY SIZE AND INTELLIGENCE

In the *Eugenics Review*, in 1953, John Nisbet opened the question of how change in family size might influence intelligence. He introduced the term "environment" as a mediating variable for the social psychological processes. He used data unparalleled for their completeness: statistics of the Scottish Education Authority based on the population of Aberdeen. The dilemma from which he started is the finding that (1) there is a consistent negative correlation between family size and intelligence; and (2) despite the plausible inference that some fraction of intelligence is inherited, there is not, through the generations, a decline in national levels. He points out that the refinement in statistical analysis implemented by keeping such factors as parental occupation or overcrowding in the home constant does not go to the central issue of contact between an adult and a child. He asserts that this exposure is inversely proportional to the size of the family, save that in large families there is a slightly higher contact for the first- and last-born children.

The premise of Nisbet's analysis is both a congenial and a familiar one. He conceives of language as the shorthand of the higher thought processes and that the ability to use language is markedly affected by the age of the child's associates.

114

The only child has a striking superiority in language development. His strategy for demonstrating the centrality of verbal exposure to adults in the development of intelligence involves three steps: (1) demonstrating a negative relationship between verbal ability and family size independent of any association with intelligence, (2) showing that the effects of family size were increased as the tests in a battery came to rely more on verbal ability, and, finally, (3) by checking the hypothesis that verbal intelligence tests applied to children at different ages would show a more marked negative effect of family size at a later age rather than at an earlier one. His data substantiated all three hypotheses—in some cases in near dramatic form. In one- or two-child families, at 11 years of age, the IQ is around 105; for seven-child families, at the same age, it is about 90. While his original paper does not take account of sociometric status, other studies indicate that in the highest occupational levels, the negative relationship between intelligence and family size virtually disappears and the highest negative correlations are found in occupations of intermediate social status.[1]

The finding that twins had lower IQ scores even though there was no tendency for them to come from larger families in Scotland provides a test of Nisbet's hypothesis which might be phrased as follows: Within any given family size, the greater the age-gap between children, the higher their intelligence. Twins, as predicted, show the lowered intelligence test performance of siblings from two-child families with short age-gaps; members of two-child sib sets with large age-gaps approximate the test performance of persons from one-child families and so forth.[2]

In summarizing her 1956 search of the literature on family, sex, and intelligence Anne Anastasi[3] concludes:

It should be noted that the psychological effect of family size on intellectual development may be curvilinear rather than

[1] John Nisbet, "Family Environment and Intelligence," *Eugenics Review* 45 (1953) 31–42.

[2] Scottish Council for Research in Education, *Social Implications of the 1947 Scottish Mental Survey* (London: University of London Press, 1953).

[3] Anne Anastasi, "Intelligence and Family Size," *Psychological Bulletin* 53 (May 1956) 187–209. Intelligence of twins may well be reduced by intra-uterine competition for available nutrition.

rectilinear. Moreover, the direction in which increasing family size influences intellectual development may itself differ with concomitant psychological and social circumstances. Attention should likewise be given to the possible effects of family size upon security, leadership, and other aspects of interpersonal relations. Available research on this question has yielded conflicting and ambiguous results. Some studies provide evidence that certain desirable emotional characteristics, as well as acceptance by associates, may be positively related to membership in relatively large families.

The data available to her were not too convincing. There was an indication relative to mutual friendships in primary grades, a finding of greater emotional security among the mentally deficient from large families.

If one were asked what size family *should* be planned in order to have intelligent children the answer from Nisbet's data would be: one-child. Failing this, one should have multi-child families only when there is a sizable age-gap between each child or, if one has a larger family he should arrange for a nanny, and later a tutor, as full-time residents in the home. With very large families older children may play these roles for younger children, but there is little evidence that tutor learns as much as tutee—so the large family still appears to leave the second to the "n-minus-one" child understimulated.

Sex-Role Identity and Adult Contact

With regard to intelligence, the direction of change desired is simple as it is in the case of biological health. One wishes to adopt practices which increase both intelligence and health, whenever this can be done without costs in other areas. With sex-role identity the matter is somewhat more complicated.

Our concept "unconscious femininity" is not to be equated with the lay construct "sissy." The qualities Teddy Roosevelt wanted to emphasize in the "outdoor life" are thought of as masculine, and there is supposed to be a positive evaluation of that style of behavior. Many conversations break down with one person attempting to tell the other that he doesn't share Teddy Roosevelt's negative evaluation of non-outdoors types, when what the conversation requires is greater consensus as to how unconsciously feminine behavior is to be described. If it did refer to men behaving like women, the referent would be clear even though it would still be hard to generalize cross-culturally. If it does not, what is a definition of potential usefulness in cross-cultural work? We were encouraged to seek such a new and potentially cross-cultural'y valid conceptualization in our own work as a result of Miller and Swanson's[4] research investigating the relationship between the selection of defenses by an individual and his unconscious and conscious sex-role identity.

Miller and Swanson used the Franck Drawing Completion Test[5] as their measure of unconscious femininity. The test is composed of 36 simple line drawings that are to be "completed" or added to as the subject desires. This process encourages the subject to organize stimuli in a manner which reveals his expressive style. Franck suggests criteria for scoring the completions. Some stimuli are to be scored only on content and others, which are quite similar, are to be scored by quite different abstract criteria. Franck permitted the use of several scoring criteria on each stimulus, and by her "multiple criteria method" a completion generally would get a unit score as feminine if it met any one of several criteria suggested as appropriate for the stimulus. This unit score would not be increased if the drawing met several of them.

In our laboratory Franck's various criteria were viewed as plausible in any given case, but it was not at all clear that any one criterion was more appropriate for one stimulus than another. For this reason all of the completions in a set of 417 protocols (obtained from a sample of second, fifth, and ninth-grade boys and girls) were scored by all of Franck's criteria and then analyzed to determine which criteria differentiated abstract drawings by boys from those by girls at each of the three grade levels.[6] After these steps, we chose 11 stimuli which, in terms of composite abstract and content

[4] Daniel Miller and Guy E. Swanson, eds., *Inner Conflict and Defense* (New York: Henry Holt, 1960).

[5] K. Franck and E. A. Rosen, "A Projective Test of Masculinity-Femininity," *Journal of Consulting Psychology* 13 (1949) 247–56.

[6] Carolyn T. Chochrane, Margaret A. Parkman, and Fred L. Strodtbeck, "The Masculinity-Femininity Model and the Prediction of Defensive Behavior in Males," unpublished manuscript.

performance, discriminated at all three grade levels. When the protocols are scored with the new, provisional scoring manual, the characterization of a completion as feminine or not corresponds relatively closely with the characterization one would make in terms of the criteria of the original Franck manual. Thus, as Franck expresses it: ". . . men expand from the stimulus outward, tend to build it up, emphasize angles, rely upon the strength of simple lines . . . . Women tend to leave the stimulus area open, elaborate within the area and draw round or blunt rather than angular, sharp lines . . . . they seem to feel a need to give support to single lines."

The second test, the Gough[7] test, is a true-false, Likert-type attitude scale based upon self-reports. The shortened version used in our research consists of a set of 24 true-false items. The subject indicates whether statements concerning culturally sex-typed preferences, interests, and attitudes are characteristic of himself. A few of the items from this test are:

I would like to be a nurse.

I very much like hunting.

I prefer a shower to a bath.

Miller and Swanson use the fact that scores on the Franck test are uncorrelated with scores on the Gough test or with other popular tests of masculinity-femininity[8] to argue that the Franck test provides a measure of "unconscious" femininity.

> If it is a test of unconscious identity, it should not correlate significantly with tests of conscious identity when administered to a large enough population. . . . It is not significantly related to any of three popular verbal tests of masculinity-femininity, the Terman-Miles Attitude Interest Analysis Test, the M-F scale of the Strong Vocational Interest Blank, and the M-F scale of the Minnesota Multiphasic Personality Inventory. Each of these three calls for reports of attitudes and interests. We felt, therefore, that Franck's test must measure something other

[7] Harrison Gough, "Identifying Psychological Femininity," *Educational and Psychological Measurement* 12 (1952) 427–39.

[8] J. C. Heston, "A Comparison of Four Masculinity-Femininity Scales," *Educational and Psychological Measurement* 7 (1948) 375–87; B. Shepler, "A Comparison of Masculinity-Femininity Measures," *Journal of Consulting Psychology* 15 (1951) 484–86.

than conscious sex identity—something which also discrimi-
nates between males and females.[9]

Our results are parallel to those of previous investigators in
that the Gough Brief Femininity Scale and the Single Criterion Franck Score are uncorrelated. Empirical evidence from
all sources is thus unequivocal on the point that the correlation between the Franck (when scored by the original or the
revised criteria) and Gough departs from zero by only an
amount which may be attributed to sampling error. However,
in our work we have taken the fact that the Franck correlated
with no other test as simply anomalous and set about to
design some related experiments which would provide more
direct support for the assumption that an "unconscious"
process was involved. These further tests[10] although not definitive were congruent with such an assumption. Hence we
follow Miller and Swanson and refer to the Franck test as the
unconscious measure and the Gough as the conscious identity
measure.

Since these two tests are uncorrelated they generate four
types: MM, MF, FM, and FF; if they are used jointly, with
cuts at the median, the first letter refers to the Franck (the
unconscious) classification.

Miller and Swanson discuss the development of sex-role
identity as follows:

> . . . each boy initially identifies with his mother and then
> transfers to his father. As an infant . . . he becomes very de-
> pendent on her because she feeds and cleans him, protects
> him from harm. . . . Later, the father usually becomes the more
> significant person. . . . He has certain unique abilities which
> the son admires. . . . By identifying with his father, a son
> gradually acquires the expressive gestures, the habits, and the
> interests that are typical of males rather than females in our
> society. We thought these earlier identifications would not be
> conscious, since they are embedded in a large number of activ-

[9] Miller and Swanson, *op. cit.* 93.
[10] Paul D. Lipsitt, "Defensiveness in Decision Making as a Function of Sex
Role Identification" (unpublished Ph.D. dissertation, University of Chicago,
1965); Margaret A. Parkman, "Identity, Role and Family Functioning" (unpublished Ph.D. dissertation, University of Chicago, 1965).

ities and occur before events are labelled verbally. Whether he is masculine or feminine in his underlying identity, the average male child, as he matures and develops friendships, feels an increasing social pressure to act in a masculine manner. . . . [These] later identifications are probably matters of conscious concern for every normal boy. They are part of his conscious sex identity.[11]

In this passage the authors make no effort to go beyond their own culture but they touch on the possibility of universal mechanisms with the thought that unconscious sex-role identity could arise in preverbal exchanges between children and their parents. They also write:

> . . . the less masculine the boy is, the earlier his developmental problems occurred. A boy with feminine identification who is relatively impervious to the meanings of his feminine traits to his peers must be fairly immature. A boy with feminine identification who wants to be masculine is more mature, since he is sensitive to the reactions of others and tries to conform. A boy with masculine identification on both levels is most mature.[12]

This argument predicts a maturity sequence $MM > FM > FF$.

In support of their formulation of the relationship between sex-role identity and selection of defenses, Miller and Swanson reported data from experimental studies. One of these by Leonard M. Lansky (Miller and Swanson, 1960) demonstrated that FF males show a significantly greater tendency, after rating nude pictures in the presence of a male experimenter, to write story endings exhibiting *denial and withdrawal*.[13] The stories involve a hero who is frustrated by a well-meaning adult to whom he is very much attached. FM males show a significantly greater tendency to write endings in which the hero expresses *aggression against the self*,[14]

[11] Miller and Swanson, *op. cit.* 89.

[12] *Ibid.* 91.

[13] An ending was scored as indicating denial if it was obviously incompatible with one of the facts in the story beginning. Withdrawal was a physical retreat from the scene of the conflict.

[14] Turning against the self was scored when the hero ignored the authority's wise counsel and suffered the consequences or if the ending described an injury to the hero.

and MM males show a significantly greater tendency to write endings in which the hero engages in *realistic problem-solving*.

To summarize the Miller and Swanson (and Lansky) studies, these authors assume that in order to withstand social pressures toward masculine identity, these pressures must either be denied or treated as if they were irrelevant to self-esteem. They assume that if such a process occurs in this area it will result in a tendency to use similar mechanisms in other situations. Thus the FF boy who denies social pressures toward masculinity will deny other social pressures. Therefore, they believe decisions made by such persons will in some sense be inferior to so-called realistic decisions. Results from a subsequent experiment[15] conducted in our laboratory has led us to reject their general formulation. We do concur with their assumption that response styles developed to deal with the core issue of the development of sex-role identity will be more generally utilized in other spheres of life, but we do not concur that MM decisions are functionally superior. To illustrate, we present the following paradigm:

The Lost Cause Experimental Design

One can use the format of a public affairs interview and rig the speeches of the specialists so that four different messages about a given problem emerge:
   A. Problem serious; individual ineffective.
   B. Problem serious; individual effective.
   C. Problem trivial; individual ineffective.
   D. Problem trivial; individual effective.
One evaluates the experiment by reading the resultant "willingness to act" of the subject. Taking into consideration the substance of the experimental tapes, one can make three plausible predictions as to the relative willingness to act of the subjects in the four cells of the design shown above.
   1. $(A + B)$ will be higher than $(C + D)$ assuming subjects are more willing to act when the problem is *serious,* i.e., $(A + B) > (C + D)$.

[15] Lipsitt, *op. cit.*

2. (B + D) will be higher than (A + C) assuming subjects are more willing to act when they believe their efforts will be *efficacious,* i.e., (B + D) > (A + C).

3. The treatment outcomes will be ordered B > A > D > C assuming (1) and (2) above are correct and *seriousness* predominates over *efficacy*; or, B > D > A > C if (1) and (2) above are correct and *efficacy* predominates over *seriousness.*

The relative weight given efficacy and seriousness is, we believe, an element of the distinction between unconscious masculinity and unconscious femininity. We believe unconsciously feminine males have identified with their mother while unconsciously masculine males have identified with their father. However, we use the term "identified with their mother" to refer to a process resulting in the incorporation of cognitive and affective orientations universally associated with the female role. How can one justify assuming the existence of near-universal communality in the cognitive-affective orientations of all women?

If one follows Guttman[16] and reasons that, save for those few women who view their work as a career or profession, women are invested in domestic and maternal roles, then the domestic-maternal milieu may be viewed as the generating mechanism for such orientations. The daily interactions of women occur in a home environment which "bears the imprint of the wishes, values, and techniques of the person central to its maintenance"—the adult female. "Within the tested and secure confines of the home, most possible and reasonable actions have already been performed, by oneself or by well-known others, and their effects are known." Moreover, developing children, unable to communicate their physical and emotional requirements, seem to require mothers who can respond intuitively to such needs. Such quick assessment precludes a rigidly maintained ego boundary and requires an intuitive responsiveness to the motivational states underlying overt behavior. Men, in contrast, daily depart from the home to confront a milieu structured by others and "in some sense their task is to impose on constantly fluctuating situations a more personal and predictable order." A persistent

[16] David Guttman, "Women and the Concept of Ego Strength," *Merrill-Palmer Quarterly* 2, no. 3 (1965) 229–40.

sense of self-other distinctions and an orientation toward assessing the likelihood that one's own goals may be realized is more likely to be generated in a milieu "in which personal ends can be achieved only by dealing with agents who have a direction, logic and structure of their own."

From this comparison, it may plausibly be suggested that the tendencies to respond intuitively to needs and to abolish self-other boundaries could be regarded as a cognitive style which develops out of women's social environment. In contrast, the tendency to detach one's subjective reactions from the processes that must be understood and to maintain a persistent sense of self-other distinctions seems better coordinated to the man's environment. In the present experiment an extrapolation from Guttman's analysis leads us to postulate that the aspect of the female complex most accessible to the FF male is just that which is involved in the contrast between the home and work environments. It is our further belief that this can be described as a tendency toward "pragmatically purposeful" versus "personally sensitive" responses rather than as "defensive" versus "nondefensive" reactions. An FF subject "personalizes" assertions, so that when he hears that the problem is a *serious* one he interprets this as likely to affect the welfare of others and hence is more quickly mobilized to act. By contrast, the task-oriented MM would be likely to defer or suppress his response to the seriousness of the situation until some recurrent and predictable structure emerges which reveals the path of effective action. A positive response to whatever was present which would constitute a demonstration of personal efficacy would be expected.

Or, stated another way, the allocentric, self-directed MM would conceive of action primarily in terms of its effects on the environment, while the autocentric, collectively-oriented FF would conceive of action primarily with regard to its effects on the people involved. Rapaport[17] has labeled these two cognitive orientations "strategic thinking" and "conscience-driven thinking." The latter arises because concern for the interpersonal effects of action leads more inevitably

[17] Anatol Rapaport, *Strategy and Conscience* (New York: Harper and Row, 1964).

to a consideration of values. Rapaport writes: "The basic question in the strategist's mind is this: 'In a conflict how can I gain an advantage over him?' The critic (conscience-driven thinker) cannot disregard the question: 'If I gain an advantage over him, what sort of person will I become?' " (p. 189).

To relate the theoretical analysis suggesting MM-FF differences in cognitive-affective style to the previous predictions of the willingness to act as a result of the treatments alone, the following systematization results. We have previously predicted that *serious* will predominate over *nonserious,* i.e., $(A + B) > (C + D)$, and *efficacy* will predominate over *nonefficacy,* i.e., $(B + D) > (A + C)$. "Predominate" here means "cause greater shift in the 'Will-act' scores." Our further analysis and theorizing enables us to relate these two earlier predictions in different ways for our two classes of subjects.

For FF's, we predict that *seriousness* is more important than *efficacy*. In the notation of the treatment cells, this is:

$$[(A + B) - (C + D)] > [(B + D) - (A + C)]$$

which reduces to

3 a) $\qquad\qquad A > D \qquad\qquad$ (for FF)

and for MM's, we predict that *efficacy* is more important than *seriousness*. In the notation used above,

$$[(B + D) - (A + C)] > [(A + B) - (C + D)]$$

which reduces to

3 b) $\qquad\qquad D > A \qquad\qquad$ (for MM)

Without taking up the details of the various experiments involved, we simply report that we have strong empirical support from two experiments that unconscious femininity predicts the selection of "lost causes" in contrast with short-run, strategic alternatives. Optimal functioning of a society requires both "impractical, theoretical, and vaguely religious thinkers" and "practical, pragmatic, and somewhat irreligious doers." The null hypothesis is simply that sex-role identity is unrelated to family size. If we find that it is related, then we will have accomplished our objective of identifying a hitherto unsuspected concomitant of the number of siblings.

FINDINGS

Our data are based upon the test responses of 373 Naval Corpsmen at Great Lakes Naval Training Station. The base frequencies are as shown in Table 1. These frequencies can be compressed together without regard for the sex ratio of

TABLE 1   Number of Siblings Plus or Minus Six Years of Subject's Age

Sisters	Brothers			
	0	1	2 or more	Total
0	30	85	47	162
1	68	44	24	136
2 or more	30	23	22	75
Total	128	152	93	373

the sibling sets to produce the distribution shown in Table 2. With regard to the Franck, the unconscious measure, there is an apparent V-relation. Boys who are only children are clearly feminine and boys from very large families are also very feminine. The trough of the V, that is, the peak of unconscious masculinity, is apparently reached by subjects from three-sibling families. This may be seen in Figure 1. There is no statistically significant evidence of there being a parabolic contour; perhaps this is due to the very much smaller frequencies in the larger family sizes. The significant difference is between the Franck and the Gough in the one-child, zero-sibling, family. Such children are more feminine by the unconscious measure and more masculine by the conscious measure.

TABLE 2   Test Scores by Number of Siblings

Siblings	Franck	Gough	N
None	5.83	8.83	30
1	5.54	9.63	153
2	5.47	9.60	106
3	5.34	9.19	41
4	5.63	10.00	24
5*	5.68	10.00	19
Total	5.53	9.56	373

* Plus three subjects with seven siblings.

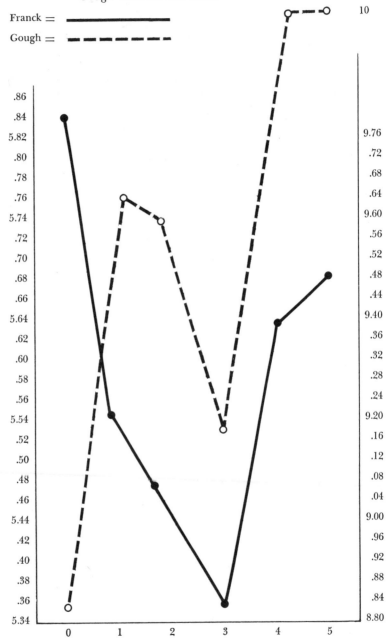

FIGURE 1 Family Size (No. of Brothers and Sisters Within (±) Six Years of Subject's Age) and Femininity on the Franck and Gough Tests for 373 Males

Franck =

Gough =

In two-child families, a boy may have a brother or a sister. Earlier work by Arthur Koch and Orville Brim indicates that the manifest femininity should be greater with the female sibling. For boys with one brother, our data disconfirm this expectation in terms of both the conscious and unconscious measures.

	Franck	Gough	N
With one brother:			
Older	5.75	10.93	32
Younger	5.66	9.52	53

For boys with one sister our data indicate unconscious masculinity and conscious femininity if the sister is older and unconscious femininity and conscious masculinity if the sister is younger.

	Franck	Gough	N
With one sister:			
Older	4.72	9.79	32
Younger	5.66	9.05	36

In the three-child family, having two sisters causes a boy to be less feminine consciously but not less feminine by the Franck measure. This may be inspected in Table 3. It may be noted that with three other siblings—this is the case which was so conspicuously masculine in Figure 1—all four patterns produce unconscious masculinity. Beyond this size our frequencies are clearly too small to investigate by differing sibling constellations. But as the total sibling set increases unconscious and conscious femininity seem to rise. This suggests that there may be an older sibling with a sufficient age-gap to serve as a parental surrogate and over-mother the younger children.

Returning to the crossover of values for zero siblings shown on Figure 1, this is a significant outlier value as judged against the differences between other corresponding values. The frequencies involved are substantial. In addition, the suggestion that in zero-sibling families FM's would be produced is highly significant in view of our other information

TABLE 3   Family Size, Sibling Constellation, and Femininity on the Franck and Gough Tests

Siblings	Average Scores		Frequencies
	Franck	Gough	
None	5.83	8.83	30
Br	5.67	9.86	85
Si	5.30	9.35	68
Br (2)	5.33	9.91	36
Br & Si	5.52	9.75	44
Si (2)	5.57	8.92	26
Br & Si (2)	5.46	9.63	11
Br (2) & Si	5.22	8.50	18
Br (3)	5.50	10.37	8
Si (3)	5.50	9.75	4
Br & Si (3)	5.70	10.20	10
Br (3) & Si	6.00	11.33	3
Br (2) & Si (2)	5.11	9.00	9
Br (4)	7.00	11.50	2
Br & Si (4)	6.00	9.00	1
Br (4) & Si	6.00	10.33	3
Br (2) & Si (3)	5.33	11.50	6
Br (3) & Si (2)	6.60	9.00	5
Br (5)	1.00	5.00	1
Br (3) & Si (4)	9.00	15.00	1
Br (2) & Si (5)	4.00	9.00	1
Br (1) & Si (6)	5.00	7.00	1
Total	5.53	9.56	373

which suggests that FM's are sometimes inappropriate in their defenses. For example, in the Lipsitt-Strodtbeck Mock Trial Experiment the guilty findings, i.e., punitive behavior against a defendant, were increased 22 per cent by FM jurors when the suggestion of homosexuality was included in the trial testimony.[18]

Table 4 shows that the 37 per cent for "no sibling" subjects exceeds by 13 percentage points the average for the other sibling sizes.

[18] Paul D. Lipsitt and Fred L. Strodtbeck, "Defensiveness in Decision-Making as a Function of Sex-Role Identification," forthcoming in the *Journal of Personality and Social Psychology*.

TABLE 4 Siblings and Sex Types

Siblings	Per cent				Base Frequency
	MM	MF	FM	FF	
None	20	17	37	26	30
One	27	24	22	27	153
Two	25	27	26	22	106
Three	27	19	27	27	41
Four +	26	18	21	35	43
Total	25	21	27	27	373

Conclusion

To retrace our argument, it appears that the heightened parental interaction in one-child families tends to promote in boys unconscious femininity as well as relatively higher intelligence. We understand unconscious masculinity to be a product of family interaction in which universalistic rules predominate. Our guess is that in very large families sex-role differentiation becomes reduced and boys become manifestly and unconsciously more feminine. In the one-child family, the conspicuous characteristic is that unconsciously feminine boys also tend to be highly masculine in their responses to the conscious test. Our data do not permit us to say with certainty how this comes about, but they do cast some doubt on the stability of Koch's earlier findings as interpreted by Brim.

LEON S. ROBERTSON
JOHN KOSA
JOEL J. ALPERT
MARGARET C. HEAGARTY

7. FAMILY SIZE AND THE USE OF MEDICAL RESOURCES*

As a part of a longitudinal study of health care among the urban poor, the Medical Care Research Unit of the Harvard Medical School is conducting studies of the utilization of medical facilities. This paper is a preliminary report on some of the findings from these studies focusing on the relationship of family size and the patterns of medical usage in this population. The results are considered to be preliminary, because data will soon be available on the medical records and morbidity of the same families from whom the data in this report were obtained. Obviously, the recall of medical visits used here are less reliable than more objectively kept medical records, and medical visits are not necessarily good indicators of morbidity.

Only a few studies have considered the relationship between family size and utilization of medical care. Stein (see reference list, item 4), using the records of a London group practice, reported no correlation between family size and the

* The research reported here was supported by grants from the U.S. Children's Bureau, Social Security Administration, Department of Health, Education and Welfare (Grant No. H-74 and H-118), and the Commonwealth Fund.

131

percentage of patients visiting the physician at least once in a year. Hare and Shaw (1) investigated the same relationship in a random sample of two English communities and found that as the number of children in the family increased, the likelihood that the parents saw a physician in a year also increased. This was true both for fathers and for mothers, but no similar correlation obtained among the children.

Although there was no relationship between family size and the proportion with at least one medical consultation among children, the average number of consultations per child decreased as family size increased. Hare and Shaw cogently pointed out that it was unlikely that the children of larger families enjoyed better health than those in small families while the parents of large families were less healthy than their counterparts in small families. Instead, they asserted, it was likely that the "strain" of managing a large family was greater than that of managing a small family. The increased stress was posited as precipitating more illness in parents which required medical attention. The decrease in average number of medical contacts for children as family size increased was probably a result of the limitations in the parents' abilities to give individual attention to each child's complaints in large families, rather than a result of better health among such children.

METHOD

The present study views the relationship of family size and use of medical facilities in a sample of 500 families who were selected from the population of users of the Medical Emergency Clinic of Children's Hospital Medical Center (Boston, Massachusetts). The sample was selected in the course of a more extensive research project on health care patterns which required that selected families live within three miles of the hospital and have no private physician who "looked after the children regularly." As a result of these criteria, the sample consisted of urban low-income families. The median income was $4,100 per year, 20 per cent were on some form of welfare, and approximately one-third of the families were Negro.

During the intake period of the program, data were collected on family size, ages of family members, and various attitudes in three home interviews with the mother. Also, in one of these interviews the mothers were asked to recall, for each family member, the number of various types of medical contacts during the year preceding the interview.

Medical contacts subsequently were classified in the following three categories:

1. visits to hospital outpatient clinic (emergency and other public clinics operated by hospitals)
2. contacts with private physician (house calls and office visits)
3. other medical contacts (well baby clinic, school health nurse or physician, home visiting nurse, polio clinic, public health nurse, guidance clinic, etc.)

RESULTS FOR PARENTS

Data on parents' use of medical facilities is available for a randomly selected 60 per cent sample of the families. Table 1 presents the average number of parental medical contacts classified by the number of children in the family and age of the parent. Among mothers under 30 years of age, the largest average number of contacts occurred for those with four or more children. However, the smallest average was found for mothers with two or three children, rather than for those with one child as one would expect on the basis of previous research. Among mothers of 30 or more years of age, there was, as expected, a considerable increase in average number of medical contacts as the number of children increased.

The types of contacts in relation to family size were also interesting. For mothers less than 30 years of age, those with larger families were less likely to report clinic visits and more likely to report private physician and other medical contacts. Mothers over 30 years of age who had large families showed an increase in clinic visits and other medical contacts and decreased consultation with private doctors when compared to those with small families. Thus, older mothers, as their families increased in size, more often relied on public facilities and less often consulted private physicians for health care.

TABLE 1   Average Number of Medical Contacts of Parents in a Year, by Age and Number of Children

	Mothers					
Age	Less than 30 years			30+ years		
No. of children	1	2–3	4+	1	2–3	4+
Clinic visits	4.15	3.83	3.59	.50	2.14	2.59
Private doctor	2.08	1.83	2.21	2.25	1.66	1.23
Other medical contacts	.75	.67	1.43	.00	.50	1.12
Total medical contacts	6.98	6.33	7.23	2.75	4.30	4.94
N	39	83	33	12	56	73

	Fathers					
Age	Less than 30 years			30+ years		
No. of children	1	2–3	4+	1	2–3	4+
Clinic visits	.74	.93	1.11	.95	1.30	1.11
Private doctor	.14	.62	.29	.30	.87	.95
Other medical contacts	.29	.13	.43	.90	.06	.20
Total medical contacts	1.17	1.68	1.83	2.15	2.23	2.26
N	28	48	14	10	61	63

The findings with respect to fathers showed the expected relationship. The larger the family, the greater the average number of total medical contacts. However, the relationship was not as strong for older fathers as it was for younger fathers. Age was an important factor taken alone in that older fathers, regardless of family size, showed a greater frequency of contacts than younger fathers, whereas the opposite was true for mothers. Furthermore, in almost every category, the rate of medical contacts for mothers was much higher than that for fathers.

One obvious possible reason for the differences between fathers and mothers was the incidence of pregnancy. However, in comparing mothers who were pregnant in the year before the interview or pregnant during the interview and mothers who were not pregnant during this time, the relationships of family size and utilization noted before were not changed appreciably. Although the average number of medical contacts was twice as frequent for pregnant mothers when compared to nonpregnant mothers, the frequency of contacts for nonpregnant mothers was about twice as high as that for fathers. The greater frequency of contacts for younger mothers was a result of more pregnancies in this group when compared to older mothers.

Since stress was hypothesized as the intervening variable between family size and the number of medical contacts, several possible indicators of stress were investigated in the analysis. These factors included the mothers' statements regarding whether the marriage was "smooth" or "upset," whether the family had more or less problems than other families, whether or not the birth of the first child was convenient, as well as three items of the Taylor Manifest Anxiety Scale (5). The items in the scale obtained the mothers' agreement or disagreement with statements regarding working under strain, tiring out quickly, and being nervous. Of these indicators, the convenience of first child's birth and the anxiety items proved to be the most useful in explaining the observed relationships.

Table 2 shows the effect of strain in the most striking way. When mothers said that they worked under strain, their medical contacts increased with family size in both age groups. On the other hand, if mothers did not agree that they worked under strain, their medical contacts decreased with increased family size. The relationships showed a similar switch when convenience of first child's birth and the other "anxiety"

TABLE 2   Average Number of Medical Contacts of Mothers in a Year, by Age, Number of Children, and Perception of Working Under Strain

Work Under Strain?	Age	Less than 30 years			30+ years		
	No. of children	1	2–3	4+	1	2–3	4+
	Clinic visits	3.15	4.21	5.54	*	1.83	3.08
Agree	Private doctor	1.25	1.81	2.00	*	2.60	1.40
	Other medical contacts	2.50	.88	2.79	*	.10	1.47
	Total medical contacts	6.90	6.90	10.33	*	4.53	5.95
	N	10	24	14	5	20	32
	Age	Less than 30 years			30+ years		
	No. of children	1	2–3	4+	1	2–3	4+
	Clinic visits	4.50	3.69	2.16	*	2.31	2.07
Disagree	Private doctor	2.36	1.84	2.37	*	1.13	.86
	Other medical contacts	.14	.58	.42	*	.72	.88
	Total medical contacts	7.00	6.11	4.95	*	4.16	3.81
	N	29	59	19	7	36	41

* N too small for averaging

items were controlled, but the degree of change was less remarkable. One may assume that the item "work under strain" was an overall indicator of stress and that more specific indicators which did not encompass all of the factors contributing to a given individual's perception of stress, therefore, had less effect.

There are also socio-cultural factors which define certain events as stressful in one context and not in another. For example, we suspected that Catholics would not perceive a large family as stressful to the same extent as Protestants. Thus, a control for religion yielded the results displayed in Table 3. The previously observed relationships were found for Protestants but not for Catholics. Protestant mothers who perceived strain had more medical contacts as family size increased, while those who did not perceive strain reported fewer medical contacts as family size increased. The differences in medical contacts by family size for Catholic mothers were much smaller and were nonlinear. There were more contacts for Catholic mothers who did not perceive strain but who had larger families than for Protestant mothers in

TABLE 3 Average Number of Medical Contacts of Mothers in a Year, by Religion, Family Size, and Perception of Working Under Strain

Work Under Strain?	Religion	Catholic			Protestant		
	No. of children	1	2–3	4+	1	2–3	4+
	Clinic visits	2.86	3.35	3.46	*	2.16	4.36
Agree	Private doctor	2.46	1.81	2.14	*	2.94	1.13
	Other medical contacts	2.27	.69	1.77	*	.83	2.00
	Total medical contacts	7.59	5.85	7.37	*	5.93	7.40
	N	11	26	26	3	16	16

Work Under Strain?	Religion	Catholic			Protestant		
	No. of children	1	2–3	4+	1	2–3	4+
	Clinic visits	2.87	3.32	2.06	5.20	3.20	2.66
Disagree	Private doctor	2.95	2.45	1.30	.90	.86	.88
	Other medical contacts	.00	.91	.92	.27	.41	.19
	Total medical contacts	5.82	6.68	4.28	6.37	4.47	3.73
	N	19	45	40	15	46	16

* N too small for averaging

136

these categories. Furthermore, Table 4 indicates that the percentage of mothers who perceived strain increased as family size increased for Protestant mothers but that among Catholic mothers there was little difference in the perception of strain with increased family size.

TABLE 4   Percentage of Mothers Who Report Working Under Strain, by Religion and Family Size

Religion		Catholic				Protestant		
No. of children	1	2–3	4+	Total	1	2–3	4+	Total
Per cent who report working under strain	37	37	39	38	17	26	50	31
N	30	71	66	167	18	62	32	112

Although no measure of fathers' perception of strain was available, the results for fathers were clarified somewhat when religion was controlled. Table 5 presents the average number of medical contacts of fathers by age, religion, and family size. The number of contacts increased as family size increased for Protestant fathers in both age groups. Catholic fathers' medical contacts decreased with family size in the older group and were related to family size in a curvilinear fashion in the younger group. These results were similar to those found for mothers.

TABLE 5   Average Number of Medical Contacts of Fathers in a Year, by Age, Family Size, and Religion

Religion

	Age	Less than 30 years			30+ years		
	No. of children	1	2–3	4+	1	2–3	4+
	Clinic visits	.81	1.04	.70	*	1.80	.85
Catholic	Private doctor	.11	.54	.40	*	1.08	1.00
	Other medical contacts	.11	.13	.20	*	.00	.14
	Total medical contacts	1.03	1.71	1.30	*	2.88	1.99
	N	18	24	10	8	33	42

	Age	Less than 30 years			30+ years		
	No. of children	1	2–3	4+	1	2–3	4+
	Clinic visits	.60	.81	*	*	.70	1.64
Protestant	Private doctor	.20	.69	*	*	.63	.90
	Other medical contacts	.60	.13	*	*	.14	.33
	Total medical contacts	1.40	1.63	*	*	1.47	2.87
	N	10	24	4	2	28	21

* N too small for averaging

137

RESULTS FOR CHILDREN

The average number of medical contacts in a year by age and number of children in the family can be seen for the children of the sample in Table 6. There was an unexpectedly larger average of total contacts for only children in both the 0-4 year and 5-9 year age groups. Secondly, the average number of total contacts decreased as family size increased in the 5-9 year age group in the same manner as in the Hare and Shaw sample. Although the average number of contacts in the 0-4 and 10-17 age groups was lowest in families of six or more children, the differences between the families with two to three and four to five children were opposite from expectation. As one would expect, the older the children, the lower the average number of medical contacts.

Examination of the data with respect to types of medical contacts revealed a tendency toward lower frequency of clinic visits as family size increased in the 5-9 year and 10-17 year age groups. There was a lower incidence of private doctor visits as family size increased in the 0-4 year and 5-9 year age groups. The tendency was toward greater frequency of other medical contacts as family size increased in the 5-9 year and 10-17 year age groups.

Because of the remarkable difference in only children and those from families of two or more children, it was decided to view the relationships with birth order controlled. These results are shown in Table 7. The average total number of medical contacts declined with family size in the 5-9 year age group in both the first- and later-born groups. However, in the 10-17 year age group the average increased as family size increased among first-born children, but the relationship was curvilinear among the later-born children. The relationships with respect to types of contacts generally were in the same direction as in the earlier table. The more pronounced increase in "other medical contacts" when family size was larger among the 10-17 year old first-borns when compared to later-borns in this age group appeared to account for the difference in the totals between these groups.

Control of the various stress indicators as perceived by

TABLE 6 Average Number of Medical Contacts per Child in a Year, by Age and Number of Children in the Family

Age	0–4				5–9				10–17			
No. of children in family	1	2–3	4–5	6+	1	2–3	4–5	6+	1	2–3	4–5	6+
Clinic visits	4.79	3.21	3.28	3.57	5.19	3.45	2.74	2.00	*	2.53	2.75	1.96
Private doctor	1.60	.73	.57	.30	1.72	.99	.34	.10	*	.13	.32	.11
Other medical contacts	3.11	2.45	2.65	2.47	.56	1.86	2.32	2.04	*	1.26	1.48	1.55
Total	9.50	6.39	6.50	6.34	7.47	6.30	5.40	4.14	*	3.92	4.55	3.62
N	80	296	141	93	16	182	205	163	5	99	157	169

* N too small for averaging

TABLE 7 Average Number of Medical Contacts per Child, by Age, Birth Order, and Number of Children in the Family

Only and First Born

Age	0–4				5–9				10–17			
No. of children in family	1	2–3	4–5	6+	1	2–3	4–5	6+	1	2–3	4–5	6+
Clinic visits	4.79	3.79	*	*	5.19	3.64	2.03	*	*	2.25	2.24	2.23
Private doctor	1.60	.94	*	*	1.72	1.07	.24	*	*	.13	.49	.22
Other medical contacts	3.11	2.50	*	*	.56	2.10	2.40	*	*	1.36	1.85	2.14
Total	9.50	7.23	*	*	7.47	6.81	4.67	*	*	3.74	4.58	4.59
N	83	70	0	0	16	101	46	6	5	61	70	54

Later Born

Age	0–4				5–9				10–17			
No. of children in family	1	2–3	4–5	6+	1	2–3	4–5	6+	1	2–3	4–5	6+
Clinic visits	**	3.03	3.28	3.57	**	3.28	2.95	2.01	**	2.99	3.17	1.83
Private doctor	**	.66	.57	.30	**	.89	.37	.09	**	.13	.18	.06
Other medical contacts	**	2.44	2.64	2.47	**	1.56	2.30	2.10	**	1.11	1.18	1.28
Total	**	6.13	6.49	6.34	**	5.73	5.62	4.20	**	4.23	4.53	3.17
N	0	226	141	93	0	81	159	156	0	38	87	115

* N too small for averaging

** Not applicable

mothers did not change the relationships of family size and per-child medical contacts.

Discussion

These findings lead to some revision of the previous interpretation of the association of family size and the use of medical resources. We have shown that, in a low-income population, increase in medical contacts for mothers as family size increased was found only for Protestant mothers who indicated that they were experiencing stress. A similar relationship held for Protestant fathers without stress controlled. Thus, it appears that the management of a large family was not perceived as stressful when the value system supported the norm that families should be large. This was the case among Catholics. For Protestants there were no such values, and the physical and mental energy required to feed, clothe, house, and care for a large family may have produced ambivalence and frustration in the parental role. However, the higher incidence of medical contacts among Catholic mothers who did not report strain may be a result of underperception of strain by Catholic mothers with larger families. The value system may not have allowed the mothers of large families to express strain, but its existence may have been manifested in medical contacts.

Whether or not stress actually increased illness or only contributed to illness anxiety is not known. The role of stress in the etiology of illness is undergoing intensive investigation at the present time, but the specific role that stress plays in the development of particular symptoms or the seeking of medical help has not been specified adequately. Nevertheless, there is general agreement that stress is an important factor in the development of many illnesses (3).

Of course, all illnesses do not come to the attention of medical personnel and our inferences about illness must be viewed in light of this fact.. Indeed, this phenomenon probably accounted for the lower number of medical contacts per child as family size increased. It may have been that only the more serious and obvious symptoms of the children came to

141

the attention of the parents when there were a large number of children. Evidence which tends to support this point was found in the pattern of medical contacts among the children studied. The increase in other medical contacts as family size increased among children five or more years of age was in contrast to the general finding. Since some of these contacts were initiated by the community rather than by parents (for example the school health nurse or physician, visiting nurse and public health nurse), the increase may have reflected a greater number of health problems which went unnoticed or were neglected by the parents of larger families and which subsequently were diagnosed by school or public health personnel.

The birth order differences suggested differential attention to children according to birth order as well as an additional speculation on the stress hypothesis. The generally greater incidence of medical contacts for only and first-born children was additional evidence for the well-documented generalization that first-borns received greater attention and extremes in treatment (2, 6) than later-borns. Although the increased medical contacts as family size increased among first-borns 10–17 years of age was not great, it was more like the trend for parents than that for the other children and suggested that these children may have had greater responsibility for the care of younger children as family size increased. Although this increased responsibility was probably not as pronounced as that of the parents, it may have been sufficiently stressful to result in symptons of which the family was more aware. Again, caution is in order because morbidity can not be inferred directly from data on use of medical resources.

SUMMARY

A sample of low-income urban families selected from users of a children's medical emergency clinic were studied. Mothers' reports of each family member's medical contacts in the year prior to the interviews were related to family size. Protestant mothers who perceived that they worked under strain showed increased medical contacts as family size increased. Either a curvilinear pattern or decrease in contacts with increased family size was found for Protestant mothers who did not report strain and for all Catholic mothers. There were, however, among mothers who did not perceive strain, more medical contacts for Catholic mothers with large families than for Protestant mothers with large families. Although a measure of perceived strain was not available for fathers, Protestant fathers were found to have increased medical contacts as family size increased. Family size made very little difference in medical contacts of Catholic fathers.

There was a general trend toward decreased medical contacts for children as family size increased. The major exception to this trend occurred in contacts other than those primarily initiated by the family for school-aged children. Contacts with school health personnel, public health nurse, and so forth increased as family size increased in this age group. With birth order controlled, oldest children over ten showed somewhat greater contacts with increased family size, a trend which was more like that of parents under strain than like that of the other children. Mothers' perception of working under strain did not affect the relation of family size and children's contacts.

It was concluded that, because the Catholics' value system supported the idea that large families were desirable, a large family was not perceived as distressful by Catholic parents. Protestant parents, not having such values, probably found the parental role more difficult as family size increased and such stress apparently increased the incidence of illness or, at least, the perception of need for medical aid. Increased medical contacts for Catholic mothers who had large families but did not perceive strain indicated the possibility of underperception of the strain of large families when the value system supported the norm that large families were desirable. The health of children in larger families may have been neglected by the parents, because the greater demand of time and energy resulted in the parents initiating fewer medical contacts for their children; hence, a greater number of problems were left to be diagnosed by school or other public health personnel. The stress of caring for younger children may have contributed to the increased contacts for oldest children over ten years of age in larger families.

REFERENCES

1. Hare, E. H. and Shaw, G. K. "A Study in Family Health: (I) Health in Relation to Family Size." *British Journal of Psychiatry* 11 (1965) 461–66.
2. Sears, R. R., *et al. Patterns of Child Rearing.* Evanston, Ill.: Row, Peterson, 1957.
3. Simmons, L. W. and Wolff, H. G. *Social Science in Medicine.* New York: Russell Sage Foundation, 1954.
4. Stein, L. "Morbidity in a London General Practice." *British Journal of Preventive and Social Medicine* 14 (1960) 9–15.
5. Taylor, Janet A. "A Personality Scale of Manifest Anxicty." *Journal of Abnormal and Social Psychology* 48 (April, 1953) 285–90.
6. Whiting, J. M. W. and Child, I. L. *Child Training and Personality: A Cross-cultural Study.* New Haven: Yale University Press, 1953.

DISCUSSION

Following is a discussion by Donald N. Barrett, Stanley Kutz, C.S.B., and Ben J. Duffy on "The Microanalysis of the Family and Fertility." Inherent in each of the four discussions is an emphasis on the need to consider the unconscious and nonrational factors which influence decisions about family size and birth control.

Mr. Barrett's discussion of Mr. Sussman's paper, "Family Inter-action and Fertility," emphasizes that birth control is not the basic issue in the discussion of fertility and population growth. Equally important are the means by which couples consciously or unconsciously make their decisions about family size. Mr. Barrett mentions the dilemma in fertility. As an example he points to the vying desires of a couple to have both a large and small family.

Similarly, Father Kutz believes that if family planning and population are to be controlled, a systematic approach to the education and liberation of influencing emotions are necessary. He says that any decision involving family size must be made objectively, taking account of the micro- and macrocosmic situation of the couple.

Mr. Barrett notes the treatment of central factors relating family size to intelligence and sex-role identity in the Strodtbeck and Creelan paper, presented at the Conference by Mr. Strodt-beck. He says that Mr. Strodtbeck "has contributed a vital effort in establishing a link in the perspectives" of demographers and sociologists. In invoking cross-discipline attention to a common problem, Mr. Barrett explains, there will be more motivation to clarify factors such as realistic problem-solving tendencies.

145

In a recap of the paper by Mr. Robertson, *et al.,* "Family Size and the Use of Medical Resources," Dr. Duffy emphasizes that medical visits are not a good indication of morbidity. Dr. Duffy also mentions the difficulty in assessing the factor of stress.

BARRETT: A survey of the research literature, focused on fertility as the dependent variable, very quickly yields the conclusion of Mr. Sussman, namely, that we know very little about the relation between family interaction and fertility. On the other hand, much certainly has been written on the subject, but credible sociological studies are few indeed. Popular articles in magazines and newspapers, such as those by Margaret Mead, often sound plausible and possibly believable, but it must be said that they are based upon idiosyncratic insights and not upon scientific research.

What Mr. Sussman has done, however, is to propose a frame of reference and to suggest lines of theoretical and experimental inquiry which would be most helpful in filling the great gaps in our knowledge. As one small illustration of this fact, it has been taken for granted that larger family sizes are prone to higher morbidity. This conclusion is based on the inference that the more complex interaction processes in the larger families promote less attention to the prevention of illness and greater facility for the spread of disease, even when income levels are held constant. It may be of interest to refer to the recent national health study which showed that the logical inferences on the relation of family size to morbidity simply were not verified.[1]

Because of the relative dearth of research evidence in contrast to the plethora of "common sense" inferences, there should be greater efforts to fill the gaps pointed out by Mr. Sussman. Two of these intervening factors need special attention. First, the focus of so much of the current discussion defines birth control as the basic issue. In a more humanly meaningful context J. Mayone Stycos (in his preface to Lee Rainwater's *And the Poor Get Children*) has observed that the issue of fertility and population growth has been viewed predominantly as a technical problem, avoiding thereby the significant processes of sexuality. The concentration of research on action programs and experimental

[1] "Selected Family Characteristics and Health Measures," Public Health Service Publication, 1,000, series 3, no. 7 (January 1967).

projects makes the understanding gained in this way simply a matter of human engineering. The fertility models developed in the Princeton Studies, the Growth of American Families Studies, and the like are more concerned about the predictability of control from one set of factors to another set than with grasping the modal pathways by which couples make these decisions, consciously or unconsciously. Birth control can hardly be a dominant goal of family life and in many cases it is rarely discussed within the context of husband-wife interaction. Effective fertility control may well include the need for large families for some and small families for others, depending on the many variables suggested in Sussman's presentation. This has applicability to less-developed as well as developed nations, as is revealed by some of the evidence we now have from Colombia. Sexuality, as conflict resolution or as part of the couple bargaining process, includes far more than engineering predictability from unimodal indexes and the like.

In a similar vein, the dilemmas of fertility require more frank exploration. In the remarkably fruitful studies of fertility in Puerto Rico by Professors Hill, Stycos, and Back, the women's expressed desire for about three children is taken as a basic grounding for the experimental program to persuade other women to limit their fertility. But the question must be asked: To what extent can we rely on this expressed desire for smaller families?

The United States studies show on the one hand that Protestants and Catholics have about the same proportions of "excess fertility," that is, basically unplanned pregnancies. On the other hand, the significant percentage of fecund couples who effectively limit their pregnancies and have fewer children than they desire has not been adequately emphasized. The attendant questions of possible frustration, disillusionment, and the like are simply not raised.

In our own studies in South America we also have found that: (1) many women realize that without control by abortion or some other method they are "procreative machines"; (2) they desire small families in the range of three or four; (3) they feel it necessary to use some effective control measures; (4) they feel their spouses agree with them in these matters (a questionable

147

response at best). At the same time, however, they realize that small families tend to be valued negatively within the context of the extended family network, about which Mr. Sussman speaks. Oscar Lewis has expressed this notion in regard to the "culture of poverty" in Mexico. Charles Wagely has shown the pride in large *parentelas* in Brazil, where large families are given positive value and support.

The primary point is that families in transitional stages of extended networks are caught in a dilemma in which they desire smaller families so that values and aspirations of human dignity can be achieved, and at the same time they desire large families which are accorded status and respect within other contexts. Our first studies show that IUD programs certainly could work effectively, but what are the responsibilities of such programs for the broader consequences for family change, stress, and crisis? Also we have found some evidence of folk abortions and even what the Population Council has called "veiled infanticide" (parents do not really try to cure seriously ill children). The medical faculties may be correct in saying that a birth control program in Colombia would be an effective way for them to discharge their duties of preventing unnecessary illnesses and deaths. But the dilemmas of couples and the dilemmas of action research programs must also be given serious attention. These remarks are certainly not made to be pessimistic about fertility and its control, but they do stress real problems demanding more knowledge.

KUTZ: I should like to explore further those parts of Mr. Sussman's paper which point to the nonrational, emotional, and unconscious elements which enter into decisions of family size and birth control. It seems that these elements have relevance not only for the microanalytic concern of the family sociologist, but for the macroanalytic concern of the demographer. It is important to understand what factors may influence couples either to exceed or fall short of the conscious goals they have set concerning family size as well as what unconscious factors may be operative in influencing couples, either individually or on a mass scale, to opt for a particular family size. In short, I think that if society is to derive the maximum benefit from the discoveries of the sociologists, these discoveries must be brought into dialogue with those of the social psychologist and the psychoanalyst.

Mr. Sussman noted that some couples utilize a logical, rationalistic mode of communication while others arrive at decisions through a more emotional, visceral mode. It should be observed that this distinction is more apparent than real. Everyone reacts and communicates emotionally, whether he knows it or acknowledges it. What passes for logical, rational communication is often a defensive cover-up for affective responses which are feared. Decisions which can be rationally and logically "justified" to oneself are often patently irrational to the unbiased observer, who can see that they do not correspond to reality. Thus, it seems to me, the real question is not whether the decision about family size is arrived at "rationally" or "viscerally," but whether it is objective, whether it really takes account of the total situation, both micro- and macrocosmic, of the couple. It would be of scant consolation to note that couples are becoming more effective in matching their actual family size with their stated objectives, if these objectives were discovered to be wildly out of proportion either with their own potential as parents or with the needs and resources of their society (which today is the whole planet).

It seems that what is required, if population is to be brought into relationship with reality, is a systematic approach to the education and liberation of the emotions. We can not tolerate much longer a situation in which decisions about family size are determined either by personal emotional distortions (for example, the need to prove masculinity by a large progeny) or by a whimsical national superego (such as the prejudice that four children—two boys, two girls—is the "in" number for the American family that is really "with it"). We must come to understand and be liberated from such unconscious determinations, for they can make decisions about family size destructive to the harmony and growth of individual couples and catastrophic for an overpopulated world.

This approach to questions of family planning and population may sound idealistic and futuristic. I can only say what I know from experience: that people who are emotionally free do make decisions which are responsible both to their family situation and to the world in which they live. I am confident that the kind of emotional liberation which can bring this objectivity will one

149

day be as normal a part of human education and development as physical fitness programs are today.

BARRETT: Without a doubt Mr. Strodtbeck has opened a Pandora's box of central factors relating family size to intelligence and sex-role identity. These connections are both important and crucial in the long history of scientific arguments about eugenics and contraception. For purposes of discussion it may be helpful to pose some different views—without averring necessarily that the proposed relations are not credible.

By reason of space and time limits, we shall not consider the fact that the "experts" are by no means unanimous on the asserted negative relation between family size and intelligence. Thomson, Burt, Fraser-Roberts, and R. A. Fisher support the thesis, but equally eminent psychologists and geneticists, such as J. B. S. Haldane, L. S. Penrose, and Lancelot Hogben, reject the evidence as proof. The British Royal Commission on Population could not come to a positive conclusion either in 1950. Nor shall we take up the problem of the appropriateness of the fundamental research tool, the intelligence test. The recent survey of Berelson and Steiner's literature shows important differences in test performance by race, sex, age, occupation and social class, national origin, birth order, and so forth. In regard to the last point, the generalization is made that, "Within families, there is a *consistent increase* in average intelligence from first-born to last-born." In a carefully controlled study, in fact, "the average advantage over the first-born rises to 18 IQ points for those born eighth or later." Perhaps, the later children have more opportunity to learn test-related skills from older siblings. Also, it could be argued whether a general intellectual factor or capacity exists.

Several methodological and interpretative questions can be raised about the Nisbet study. It is quite true that many studies, using a variety of instruments applied to widely diverse groups, have shown almost without exception a small but unquestionably significant negative correlation between number of siblings and intelligence scores of school-age children—with coefficients ranging from about −.2 to −.3. However, use of some of these data raises serious questions. A sample of 11-year-old children in a population such as Aberdeen, Scotland can be given intelligence tests and family size data can be obtained. But the IQ of an 11-year-old may have no relation to the IQ's of other family members, siblings included. In fact, many researchers have pointed to well-established positive correlations between mates and relatives, even where a negative relation between IQ and family size seems evident. Further, a given 11-year-old may be a first-born, a third-, or a tenth-born in families where pregnancies occurred very close together or were widely spaced. Since there is some evidence of a lengthening of the fecundity period, it may be pointed out that a woman marrying at age 20 can space children three years apart and still have eight to ten children.

The Scottish Mental Survey Committee resurveyed the entire group of 11-year-olds in Scotland in 1947 (70,000 subjects) for comparison with a similar study done in 1932. They report the familiar inverse correlation between intelligence and family size, but they also found the 1947 mean test score to be about two IQ points higher than the 1932 mean. No evidence is given for the lame explanation that this is due to increase in test sophistication. Even if the environmental explantion is correct, why could it not also be better nutrition, even for the larger family sizes? Findings of increased test scores have also occurred in New Zealand, in Leicester-Devonshire, and a survey of English school districts.

The point to be made here is simply that Nisbet's study is provocative but does not stand alone in scientific circles. Solid conclusions are difficult at best.

Mr. Strodtbeck's own research into sex-role identity and adult contact explores an area in which demographers and sociologists have been notably absent. This can not be explained by the proclivity of the social psychologist to do laboratory studies and the sociologist to do survey research. The "Lost Cause" experimental design is applied to Naval Corpsmen in a fundamentally creative way.

In 1942, Flanagan used the Bernreuter Personality Inventory and uncovered little evidence of any association between personality characteristics and measures of fertility. The Indianapolis study of the socio-psychological factors affecting fertility yielded relatively few significant factors. Some evidence was uncovered in an extensive and longitudinal set of studies that women had

151

fewer children who showed tendencies toward introversion, sub-missiveness, inferiority, and poor emotional and social adjust-ment. The correlations average about .20. At the same time the Indianapolis data show that emotionally stable women control the number and spacing of pregnancies more effectively. In the Princeton study of two-child families, the researchers with the aid of psychologists developed and applied tests of eight person-ality characteristics to their sample of respondents. Of ten hypoth-eses tested, only three reached statistically significant levels related to number of children desired: anxiety, compulsiveness, and ambiguity tolerance. Even these account for only 1 per cent of the total variance of the number of children desired. The latter, however, was the most significant factor in predicting actual fertility.

In turn, family sociologists have tended to discriminate the sexuality component in terms of empirically ascertained differ-ences between men and women. There seems to be general agree-ment, for example, that men and women, as categories but not always as individuals, differ on the following: sexual activity before marriage, general premarital attitude toward sex, pre-ferred frequency of intercourse, satisfaction from intercourse, frequency of orgasm, and frequency of refusal to have intercourse.

These research experiences and orientations, then, help to ex-plain the absence of involvement by demographers and sociolo-gists in such an important area as testing the relations between family size, sibling positions, and masculinity-femininity meas-ures. Mr. Strodtbeck has contributed a vital effort in establishing a link in the perspectives. Demographers may appear dubious as to the cross-national and even one-nation meaning of "femininity" and the measures thereof, but when, as Mr. Strodtbeck points out, this factor can be related significantly to family sib-composition variations, a common interest is provoked. Another step in this process of bringing about cross-discipline attention to a com-mon problem consists in more clarification of such factors as "leadership" styles in the personality-family configuration, "re-alistic problem-solving" tendencies, and the like.

Of particular value in Mr. Strodtbeck's approach are the con-siderable number of openings for further inquiry. The cross-cultural problem of masculinity-femininity measurement as related to family size has already been mentioned and has solidly provoked the question of similar effort for our studies in South America. But the more specific interactional meaning of family size in terms of selected family composition sets (differentiated not only by sex, but by age, family cycle stage, and the like) sheds new light on the need for deeper inquiry. This is the test for fruitful research.

DUFFY: Mr. Leon S. Robertson and his associates have provided us with the preliminary results of a study which seeks to relate family size, patterns of medical use, and the occurrence of stress in the parents of the families studied. It must be emphasized, as the authors state, that medical visits are not a good indication of morbidity. Actually, medical visits vary with their availability, patient understanding and motivation, and the degree of development of the community. The more developed the medical care program, the more visits are recorded per family. Utilization varies directly with the organization of the service.

Stress is an extremely difficult factor to assess. We do not yet have any biochemical indicator or test, and the socio-psychological analyses are essentially descriptive and not quantitative. It is impossible to say anything meaningful about stress equivalents in the present state of knowledge.

A more intensive study of family size and utilization of health services is possible with the newly developed neighborhood health center concept. Such a health center has been established in a Boston urban poverty area by the Department of Preventive Medicine at Tufts University Medical School. Briefly, this is a comprehensive medical and social service center which operates seven days a week and 24 hours a day.

There are no barriers of accessibility or income size. The center is within the community and the services, to a housing project-welfare population of 1,200 families, are provided without charge.

The treatment unit is the family health care team of internist, pediatrician, public health nurse, and social worker. Community health aides and family development workers recruited from the community are being trained. The objective will be to render an integrated, family-centered type of health care.

It will be possible to study the question of family structure

153

and utilization of services and begin to develop some quantitative ideas of the multiple factors that determine family well-being. The valuable contributions of the Harvard study can be further tested in a defined population subjected to intensive study and, it is hoped, a continuing process of involvement in self-improvement, family strengthening, community organization, and social change.

PART FOUR

Values, Technology, and Family Planning

CHARLES F. WESTOFF
NORMAN B. RYDER

8. METHODS OF FERTILITY CONTROL IN THE UNITED STATES: 1955, 1960 AND 1965 *

The 1965 National Fertility Study provides the opportunity to examine changes over a decade in the methods of fertility control employed by married couples in the United States, because its design is comparable with those of the surveys conducted in 1955 and again in 1960.[1] Three circumstances make such an examination especially interesting at this time. First, the birth rate has been declining since 1957; this change cannot be explained without analysis of fertility regulation. In the second place, the oral contraceptive has recently emerged as a leading method of birth control.[2] Thirdly, the

* The paper is based upon data collected in the 1965 National Fertility Study under a contract with the National Institute of Child Health and Human Development. The authors would like to acknowledge the able assistance of Susan Hyland of the Office of Population Research, Princeton University, who was responsible for the data processing.

[1] The principal reports of these studies are: Ronald Freedman, Pascal K. Whelpton, and Arthur A. Campbell, *Family Planning, Sterility and Population Growth* (New York: McGraw-Hill, 1959); Pascal K. Whelpton, Arthur A. Campbell, and John E. Patterson, *Fertility and Family Planning in the United States* (Princeton, N.J.: Princeton University Press, 1966).

[2] Norman B. Ryder and Charles F. Westoff, "Use of Oral Contraception in the United States, 1965," *Science* 153, no. 3741 (September 9, 1966) 1199–1205.

Catholic Church is currently reviewing its position on the subject of birth control.

COMPARABILITY OF THE SURVEYS

All three of the national sample surveys collected data for white married women, ages 18–39, husband present. The coverage of the 1960 study also included Negro women, and the upper age limit was extended to 44. The 1965 study provided a double sample of Negro women and enlarged the age span further to include all married women, husband present, born since July 1, 1910. The data presented in this paper, however, cover only women 18–39 from all three surveys.

In some respects the data included here are not completely comparable over time. In both 1955 and 1960, the methods of contraception ever used were determined by responses to a single general question on use; in 1965, the question was asked specifically for each separate interpregnancy interval and methods *ever* used were estimated by summing over all intervals. This change was introduced with the intention of increasing the accuracy of report; the consequence may have been to increase the incidence of methods used, at the expense of comparability. Another particular difference was a modification of the way in which information was obtained concerning the practice of douching for contraceptive purposes. A third difference was the ordering of options on the card to which the respondent was referred in replying to the question about methods used; it is suspected that a changed order is responsible for the substantial report of abstinence as a method in 1960 but not in 1955 or 1965. A fourth small difference is that age was defined in 1955 and 1960 as age at time of interview, but in 1965 as age at midyear, 1965; in consequence, the women in 1965 are some four or five months older, on the average, than the women in the previous two surveys. Finally, the surveys of 1955 and 1960 were conducted by the Survey Research Center, University of Michigan, while the survey for 1965 was conducted by National Analysts, Inc.,

Philadelphia. Differences between these organizations in procedures for obtaining a national sample do not appear to have affected comparability. With these exceptions then, the estimates for comparisons through time would appear to be reliable within the limits of sampling variability.

METHODS EVER USED

It is of some importance for interpretation of the results of this paper, which refer to using couples, that the proportion of couples reporting that they had ever used contraception[3] rose between 1960 and 1965, continuing a trend observed between 1955 and 1960. The increase is most evident among those who had the lowest rates of reported use—the nonwhites, the Catholics, and the younger women. The general trend of fertility regulation will be the subject of another report; the focus here is on the different methods of fertility control reported by users.

Between 1955 and 1960 the number of methods per using couple increased by nearly 10 per cent (from 1.70 to 1.86); two methods showed statistically significant increases—condom, and jelly (alone). By 1965 the number of methods per using couple had increased to 1.98, perhaps in part because of the change in survey procedure already noted, but almost certainly also because of the availability of a new method, the oral contraceptive.

It is apparent from Table 1 that there has been a major change in the use of various methods between 1960 and 1965. For whites and nonwhites alike, the use of rhythm, diaphragm, and condom decreased sharply in favor of the oral contraceptive. First licensed for contraceptive prescription in June, 1960, use of the pill has risen at an increasing rate; by the time of our interviews in late 1965, 33 per cent of white

[3] Couples are classified as using contraception on a motive basis rather than on an action basis. This procedure excludes behavior which is contraceptive in effect but not in stated intent, such as the use of the pill for medical reasons only. The extent of the latter activity is not insignificant, particularly for Catholics. (See Ryder and Westoff, *op. cit.* 1200.) To the extent that there is dissimulation about reasons for using the pill, the estimates of use of oral contraception reported in the present paper are understated.

TABLE 1 Percentage of Users Who Have Ever Used Specified Method of Contraception, by Color and by Religion of White Wives 18–39, 1955, 1960, and 1965

| | White | | | | | | | | | | | | Nonwhite[1] | |
| | Total White | | | Protestant | | | Catholic | | | Jewish | | | | |
Method	1955	1960	1965	1955	1960	1965	1955	1960	1965	1955	1960	1965	1960	1965
Number of users	1,901	1,948	2,445	1,362	1,347	1,648	453	466	655	64	101	55	160	651
Percentage reporting:*														
Condom	43	50	42	48	56	45	25	28	28	72	74	67	58	43
Rhythm	34	35	31	25	27	21	65	67	59	8	9	13	18	11
Pill	—	—	33	—	—	36	—	—	25	—	—	25	—	29
Douche	28	24	28	32	28	32	18	17	20	11	8	14	50	53
Diaphragm	36	38	26	41	46	31	17	12	11	56	51	45	30	17
Withdrawal	15	17	15	17	18	15	13	17	15	6	4	9	21	14
Jelly alone	6	11	9	8	14	11	2	4	4	2	8	2	19	19
All other	8	11	14	12	12	17	4	12	8	3	2	2	19	35
Total[2]	170	186	198	183	201	209	144	157	169	158	156	177	215	219

* Percentages have been rounded off in all cases.

[1] The 1955 sample was confined to the white population.

[2] The total exceeds 100 because many couples reported two or more methods ever used.

Source: Percentages for 1955 and 1960 adapted from Whelpton, Campbell, and Patterson, op. cit., Table 156, page 278, and Table 196, page 360.

FIGURE 1 Percentage of Users Who Have Ever Used Specified
Method of Contraception (Whites), 1955, 1960 and 1965

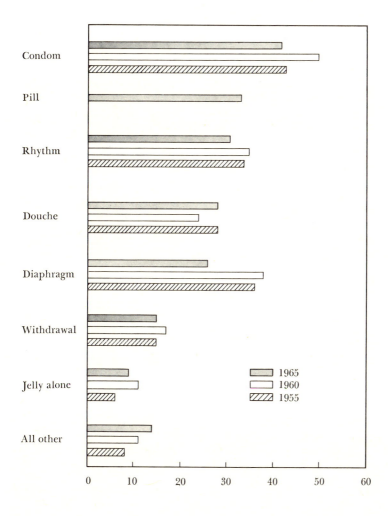

women and 29 per cent of nonwhite women ever using any
method reported having used the pill. It seems that the pill
has been adopted primarily by couples who would otherwise
have used, or were formerly using, the diaphragm, the condom, or the rhythm method. Although the douche shows an

161

FIGURE 2 Percentage of Users Who Have Ever Used Specified Method of Contraception (Nonwhites), 1960 and 1965

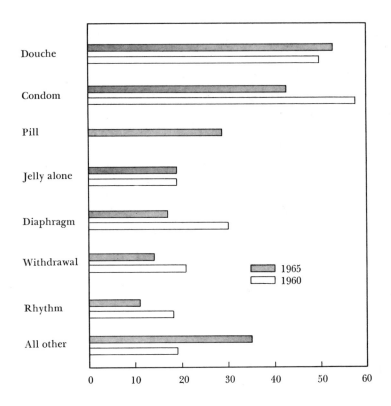

apparent increase in use, the change is probably artifactual.[4]

The residual category of "all other" methods is comprised principally of suppositories, foam, and the intra-uterine contraceptive device. The last of these, which did not become generally available until 1964, is reported as a method used by 1.3 per cent of white users and by 2.8 per cent of non-

---

[4] Douching may be used for personal hygiene as well as for contraception. The reported figure refers only to women who asserted contraceptive intent. Furthermore, douching is frequently a supplementary technique to other methods of contraception. Much of the use reported in this paper involves techniques employed in combination.

white users. These proportions may be expected to increase considerably in the years ahead. Suppositories were employed by 6 per cent of white users and by 16 per cent of nonwhite users in 1960; the proportions were approximately the same (5 per cent and 17 per cent respectively) in 1965. Use of the vaginal foam method was insignificant in 1960, but by 1965 the method had been employed by 7 per cent of white users and by 15 per cent of nonwhite users.

There are some important differences in the patterns of change in methods used among the major religious groupings of the white population. The methods most used by Protestant couples in 1955 and in 1960 had been the condom and the diaphragm; both declined substantially by 1965. Reliance on the condom and the diaphragm was even more pronounced among Jewish couples; by 1965 use of both had declined but less so than for Protestants, and use of the pill is less frequent than for Protestants.

Among Catholic women the picture of change is dominated by the appearance of the pill between 1960 and 1965. The number of methods used per couple has increased from 1.57 to 1.69 and there has been a decrease in the proportion reporting that they have ever used the rhythm method. "Abstinence" as a method was reported by 9 per cent of women using any method in 1960, and by less than 1 per cent in 1965; the difference is probably attributable to the change of salience of the method in the questionnaire format.

CHANGES IN METHODS MOST RECENTLY USED

In Table 1, the methods described are those which the respondents have *ever* used. In consequence, the experience reported may extend, for some of the women, back over 25 years prior to the date of interview. In order to examine the most recent behavior of the samples, Table 2 has been prepared. It differs from Table 1 in that the methods are those used most recently; in temporal terms the appropriate comparison is between the techniques of fertility control employed by American couples during the first half of the 1950's and those of a decade later. A further difference between

163

Tables 1 and 2 is that whereas methods *ever* used are described in Table 1—and thus many couples are included more than once—each couple is represented only once in the distributions of Table 2. The data for 1960 are omitted because the procedures followed in 1960 do not permit comparability.[5] While the bases for the 1955 and 1965 estimates are not exactly the same[6] they are more alike than either is with the 1960 study.

The impact of the pill on the distribution of methods used is revealed more clearly in the data on methods most recently used than in the comparison of methods ever used. Reliance on the condom, the diaphragm, and rhythm—which, in terms of separate use, amounted to 74 per cent in 1955—had declined to 41 per cent by 1965. The pill, which is responsible for this change, has now become the most popular method of contraception used by American couples, a fact that would be even more pronounced if the comparisons were restricted to the younger women in the sample. The method showing the greatest concomitant decline is the diaphragm, followed by the rhythm method and the condom.

The patterns of change are not the same for couples of different religions. Among couples with Protestant wives, use of the diaphragm and condom have declined appreciably and use of the rhythm method has virtually disappeared. The pill now clearly dominates the picture as the most popular method.

The patterns of change for Jewish couples seem reasonable, although the numbers in the two studies are quite small. As with Protestants, both the condom and diaphragm have declined in popularity with the adoption of the pill, but both methods continue to be used by Jewish couples much more extensively than by others. Thus 71 per cent of Jewish couples still depend on these two mechanical methods compared

[5] In 1960 the respondents were not queried about which method they used last if they were alternating use among two or more methods.

[6] In the 1965 study, unlike the 1955 investigation, the respondent who last used a method in an interval prior to the last pregnancy was not asked which method was used last if the couple used methods alternately. As a result, a higher proportion of couples interviewed in 1965 are classified in the category "Other Multiple Methods."

164

TABLE 2   Methods of Contraception Used Most Recently, by Religion of White Wives 18–39, 1955 and 1965

Method	Total White[1]		Protestant		Catholic		Jewish	
	1955	1965	1955	1965	1955	1965	1955	1965
Number of users:[2]	1901	2445	1362	1648	453	655	64	55
Per cent total:	100	100	100	100	100	100	100	100
Pill	—	24	—	27	—	18	—	22
Condom	27	18	30	19	15	15	56	44
Rhythm	22	13	12	4	54	36	2	—
Diaphragm	25	10	29	12	12	4	37	27
Douche	8	6	9	7	4	4	—	—
Withdrawal	7	5	7	5	8	7	3	—
Jelly alone	4	2	5	3	—	1	2	—
Other single methods	2	6	2	7	1	4	—	—
Condom and douche	1	3	1	3	1	2	—	—
Pill and any other	—	3	—	3	—	2	—	2
Rhythm and douche	2	2	2	1	3	2	—	2
Other multiple methods	2	8	3	9	2	5	—	4

[1] Totals include white women of other religions.

[2] Includes a small number of women who reported using contraception but for whom specific method is unknown.

Source: The 1955 data were tabulated in a slightly different form in Christopher Tietze, "The Current Status of Contraceptive Practice in the United States, "*Proceedings of the Rudolf Virchow Medical Society*, vol. 19, 1960, page 30.

with only 31 per cent of Protestants and 19 per cent of Catholics.

Among couples with Catholic wives, the major change has been a decline in reliance on the rhythm method—from 54 to 36 per cent. The extent of use of the condom has not changed, but the diaphragm has declined in use from 12 to 4 per cent. The pill appears to have become the second most popular method of fertility control among Catholic couples.

CATHOLIC CONFORMITY

Although reliance on the formally accepted rhythm method is still the most common contraceptive practice by 1965, nearly two-thirds of the Catholic women who report having used some method of fertility control have at some time employed practices inconsistent with traditional Church doctrine, a position which, although under review by ecclesiastical authorities, has at this writing not been changed.

FIGURE 3   Method of Contraception Used Most Recently by White Women, 1955 and 1965

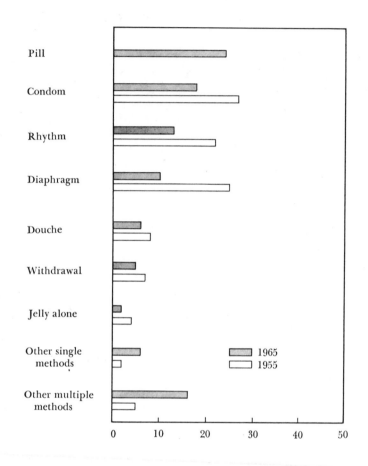

Since the data presented thus far are restricted to those who report use of some method of fertility regulation and since Catholics who use no method are also conforming to doctrine, an assertion about conformity requires consideration of the behavior of all Catholic women. Table 3 therefore includes all Catholic women, as well as those who reported ever having used a method. It should be emphasized that this analysis reverts to the concept "ever used"; although it

TABLE 3 Percentage of Catholic Women Conforming to Catholic Doctrine on Contraception, by Frequency of Church Attendance, 1955, 1960, and 1965

Year and Frequency[1] of Church Attendance	All Catholic Women						Catholic Women Ever Using Any Method	
	Number of women	Per cent total	Total conformed	Non-users	Used rhythm only	Used other methods	Number of women	Per cent using rhythm only
Total								
1955	787	100	70	43	27	30	453	47
1960	668	100	62	30	31	38	466	45
1965	843	100	47	22	25	53	655	32
Regular								
1955	533	100	78	45	33	22	293	60
1960	525	100	69	32	37	31	357	54
1965	607	100	56	23	33	44	468	43
Less frequent								
1955	254	100	53	40	13	47	152	22
1960	143	100	35	25	10	65	107	13
1965	236	100	26	21	5	74	186	6

[1] "Regular" means "regularly" in the 1955 and "once a week" in the 1960 survey in reference to questions on the frequency of attendance at religious services. In the 1965 survey the category means "once a week or more" to a question on attendance at Mass.

Source: Percentages for 1955 and 1960 adapted from Whelpton, Campbell, and Patterson, *op. cit.*, Table 160, page 285.

includes recent behavior it is not confined to the immediate past.

The proportion of all Catholic women who have attempted to regulate their fertility by use of the rhythm method exclusively has changed only a little between 1955 and 1965 (from 27 per cent to 31 per cent to 25 per cent); meanwhile the proportion using no method has declined from 43 per cent to 30 per cent to 22 per cent. In consequence, the proportion not conforming (in this sense) has increased from 30 per cent to 38 per cent to 53 per cent. In 1965 a majority of married Catholic women aged 18–39 reported having used methods inconsistent with the traditional Church doctrine on birth control.

Individuals differ widely, of course, in their adherence to religious values and church requirements and, among Catholics at least, such variation is associated with contraceptive behavior. To assess the significance of this dimension for the change over the years we include in Table 3 a simple breakdown of Catholic respondents by whether they attend church regularly or not.[7] As expected, the proportion conforming varies directly with the frequency of attendance. The more interesting observation, however, is that for both categories of attendance the trend over time is toward nonconformity. And this generalization holds regardless of whether the comparisons are based on all Catholic women or only on those who reported ever having used some method of family limitation.

There is an understandable temptation to infer that the trend toward nonconformity among Catholic women is a response to the deliberations of Church officials about fertility regulation, reflecting confusion in the public mind about the possibility of change in the official position. Although this may be part of the explanation of the acceleration in the decline of conforming behavior between 1960 and 1965, it does not seem satisfactory as a complete explanation of the change, because it represented a continuation of a trend already observed between 1955 and 1960. Furthermore, the acceptance of oral contraception, which is

---

[7] Additional more refined measures of religiousness are available in the 1965 study and will be included in subsequent reports.

principally responsible for the increase in nonconforming behavior among Catholics between 1960 and 1965, is paralleled by an even greater adoption of the pill by nonCatholics. The most significant finding of our study to date has been the increase in the use by married couples of fertility regulation in general and oral contraception in particular, a proposition that holds for Catholics and nonCatholics alike.

NORMAN B. RYDER
CHARLES F. WESTOFF

9. ORAL CONTRACEPTION AND AMERICAN BIRTH RATES*

Since 1957 the birth rate has fallen by more than one quarter after a decade on a high and even slightly ascending plateau. The postwar movements of the crude birth rate are shown in Figure 1. The primary purpose of this paper is to explain these changes. To this end, we present here two relevant types of inquiry: first, an assessment of the purely demographic characteristics of postwar reproductive behavior, based on official vital statistics, and second, a preliminary appraisal of the extent to which use of the oral contraceptive may have been responsible for the observed change, based on data from the 1965 National Fertility Study.

I. The Birth Rate and Total Fertility Rate

The first step is to remove the influence of the changing age distribution on the time series of the birth rate. The birth rate is the product of the rates at which women of vari-

* This paper is based in part on data collected in the 1965 National Fertility Study under a contract with the National Institute of Child Health and Human Development. The authors would like to acknowledge the able assistance of Susan Hyland of the Office of Population Research, Princeton University, who was responsible for the processing of data from the 1965 study.

171

ous ages are bearing children and the proportional representation of those women in the total population. The
conventional way of deriving fertility movements which are
independent of changes in the age distribution is to calculate for each year a total fertility rate, the sum of the birth
rates for women of each individual age. The result of this
operation is also presented in Figure 1.[1] Clearly something
other than the evolving age distribution must be responsible
for the observed decline: the birth rate has gone down by 27
per cent and the total fertility rate by 26 per cent since 1957.

But there is some reward from the examination of the
series for the more refined index. In the first place, we see
that the high plateau for the birth rate was a delusion produced by the changing age distribution. From 1950 to 1957
the total fertility rate was climbing by 23 per cent while the
crude birth rate rose by only 6 per cent. The influence of the
fertility level on the birth rate was largely negated by a progressive decline in the representation of women in the reproductive ages, itself an echo of our depression experience.
Thus the location of the high fertility plateau is more properly the 1956–61 period. In the second place, the decline
which it is our principal charge to explain is that from 3620
in 1961 to 2754 in 1966, a drop of 24 per cent in five years.[2]
It is interesting, finally, to note that the birth rate has
declined less in the 1961–65 interval than the total fertility
rate—the age distribution has recently started to become more
favorable for reproduction.

II. The Translation of Total Fertility

There are two sources of variation from year to year in the
total fertility rate: (1) changes in the amount of completed

[1] All of the fertility rates used in this paper are taken from Table 3 of
Pascal K. Whelpton and Arthur A. Campbell, *Fertility Tables for Birth
Cohorts of American Women,* Vital Statistics—Special Reports 51, no. 1 (Jan-
uary 29, 1960) 1–129 (U.S. National Office of Vital Statistics); and from Tables
1–18 of *Vital Statistics of the United States, 1964,* vol. 1: *Natality* (U.S. National
Center for Health Statistics).

[2] The crude birth rate for 1966 has been estimated at 18.6 on the basis of
provisional totals for the first ten months. The total fertility rate for 1966 has
been estimated at 2754 by assuming that the trend in the ratio of the total
fertility rate to the crude birth rate, 1961–65, continues in 1966.

FIGURE 1 Crude Birth Rate (C.B.R.) and Total Fertility Rate (T.F.R.) United States, 1946–66

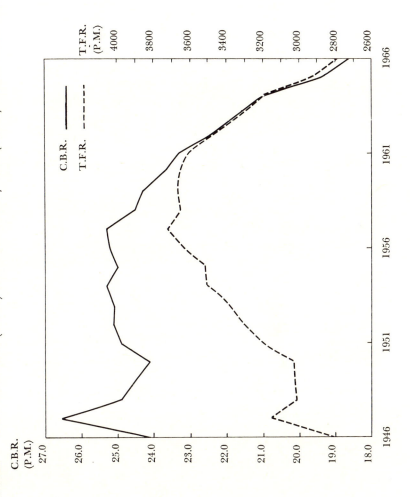

173

fertility achieved by women in successive cohorts, (2) changes in the time pattern of childbearing from cohort to cohort. The explanation for the second source of change is roughly as follows: If successive cohorts bear their children at progressively earlier ages, there is a more than ordinary overlap of their fertility in any one year, and the period total fertility rate is distorted upward while the change is under way; if there is a progressive delay of childbearing, there is conversely a temporary downward distortion.

A formula has been devised to correct for the distortion attributable to time pattern changes which yields translated total fertility rates.[3] The procedure is this: The formula for estimating the amount of cohort fertility (F^*) on the basis of the amount of period fertility (F) and the annual change in the mean age of period fertility (A) is: $F^* = F(1+A)$. For present purposes we have considered separately the age-specific birth rates of each order.[4] Separately for 1955–59 and 1960–64, and for each order of birth, we have calculated the mean total fertility rate and the per annum change in the mean age of fertility. Then, to get a translated total fertility rate for each of the two periods, we have summed the results over all orders. (See Table 1.) We find that the observed total fertility rate declined from 3640 to 3455 between 1955–59 and 1960–64, but the translated total fertility rate actually rose from 3258 to 3595 in the same interval.[5] Put in other terms, there was positive distortion of 11.7

[3] Norman B. Ryder, "The Process of Demographic Translation," *Demography* 1 no. 1, (1964) 74–82.

[4] Individual orders of birth have been used to improve the probability that the observed behavior will correspond with the assumptions on the basis of which the formula was developed, specifically to reduce variance in the age distribution of fertility and to reduce the curvature of the time series.

[5] These measures show what the period total fertility rate would have been had there been no change in the time pattern of fertility from cohort to cohort. They do not represent estimates of the level of cohort fertility, because each component order-specific total has its own temporal location. Any period total fertility rate is a combination of the lower-order childbearing of later cohorts and the higher-order childbearing of earlier cohorts. If, as has happened recently in the United States, there is a tendency on the one hand for more lower-order fertility combined with a tendency for less higher-order fertility from cohort to cohort, the consequence is an inflation of the period total fertility rate (aside from changes in the time pattern of childbearing) over the corresponding cohort level.

per cent (caused by a trend toward younger childbearing) in the 1955–59 period and negative distortion of 1.4 per cent (caused by a trend toward older childbearing) in the 1960–64 period, converting a real increase of 7.6 per cent into an apparent decrease of 5.1 per cent.

TABLE 1   Observed and Translated Order-specific Total Fertility Rates, United States, 1955–59 and 1960–64

| | Observed | | Translated | |
	1955–59	1960–64	1955–59	1960–64
I	1009	888	922	986
II	957	837	820	836
III	704	664	618	679
IV	419	436	386	448
V	229	257	219	265
VI	129	149	124	156
VII	75	88	69	90
VIII+	118	136	100	135
Total	3640	3455	3258	3595

As one way of making more plausible this apparently perverse finding, consider the actual childbearing of the 1931 cohort, which was the mean cohort represented in the childbearing of 1955–59, and of the 1936 cohort, which was the mean cohort of the 1960–64 period. The younger cohort is at age 31.0 at the end of the available time series (the end of 1966) and it has a cumulated fertility rate estimated at 2767. When the 1931 cohort was at the same age, its cumulated fertility rate was only 2588. Thus the rise in fertility obtained by translation seems to reflect accurately the changes in cohort performance which underlie the period-specific data.

Our assertion on the basis of these data is that the decline in the total fertility rate from 1957 to the present is not so much a reflection of decline in the mean completed parity of cohorts, as it is a consequence of a large transformation of the time pattern of childbearing, from a progressively earlier pattern in the 1950's to a progressively later pattern in the 1960's. The data, order by order, show a persistent decline in the mean age of births of each order (totaling two years of age on the average) for the period 1946-62, followed by a

175

sharp rise since 1962. The empirical change which most requires explanation is the modified time pattern; changes in the level of fertility seem secondary, at least within the range of these data.

It is important to emphasize that nothing in the data at hand precludes the possibility that wives who are now in an early phase of family formation may eventually have fewer children than their predecessors. Indeed, as a general rule, women who bear children later eventually have fewer children. Other data from the National Fertility Study concerning the future intentions of the women in our sample will give us some basis for assessing the probability of a reduction in mean completed parity.

III. The Timing of Marriage

Our analysis of order-specific fertility rates leads to the conclusion that most of the year-to-year movement in total fertility recently has been a reflection of changes in the time pattern of childbearing. Since these rates are based on women of all marital statuses, they reflect the level and timing of nuptiality as well as of marital fertility. It is accordingly appropriate to consider the evidence on recent changes in age at marriage.

It is difficult to study nuptiality in the United States, because the data required for responsible analysis are either incomplete (registration data) or subject to various inaccuracies (enumeration data). Using the best information available, Arthur A. Campbell has produced estimates of first marriage rates by single ages and single years for the years through 1961. Using similar procedures, we have continued these estimates through 1964. The results of this inquiry are as follows: The mean age of women at first marriage declined sharply in the postwar period to a level of approximately 21.4, at which it remained during 1950-59. Meanwhile, the mean age of women at the time of their first birth declined from 23.2 to 22.4, indicating an important independent change, namely, a shortening of the interval between marriage and first birth. In the 1960's the mean age at marriage has risen, from 21.3 in 1961 to 21.7 in 1964. The rise in the mean age at first birth has been more limited and more recent, as would be expected from a lagged phenomenon. Its minimum was not reached until 1963 (22.2); in 1964 it was 22.4. At this time, at least until the 1965 and 1966 data are in, it is not possible to assert that anything is happening to the time pattern of first order fertility that could not be attributable to the rise in the mean age at first marriage.

By independent procedures, the Bureau of the Census has prepared estimates of *median* age at first marriage, from data collected in their current population surveys. This value was 20.2 for the years 1952-59 and has since risen to 20.5 in 1964 and 20.6 in 1965.[6] This is the same pattern as described above for mean ages at first marriage. The question about the relation between marriage changes and fertility changes is approached from a different standpoint in Section V.

IV. The Oral Contraceptive Calendar

The second part of our paper is concerned with the question of possible relationships between the decline in fertility during the 1960's and the rise in the use of oral contraception during the same period. It is our intention to investigate subsequently the links between contraceptive behavior and reproductive behavior on an individual basis; the present analysis is confined to some macroanalytic comparisons.

Because we were interested in capturing the early history of dissemination of the oral contraceptive, we asked all women who reported any use of the pill to tell us in which months they had used it, for the period since January, 1960. These data permit us to calculate, month by month, the proportion of women using the pill—a unique time series of considerable interest not only in relation to fertility movements per se but also to the broader study of the diffusion of innovations.

The appropriate base for each month's proportion was determined by ascertaining the number of respondents who

[6] U.S. Bureau of the Census, *Current Population Reports,* series P-20, no. 144 (November 10, 1965).

had been first married prior to the date concerned. Our numerators are inflated a little by the assumption that all reported pill use occurred subsequent to marriage; on the other hand the denominators are also inflated a little by the assumption that all of these women remained married. Neither of these biases is likely to be more than trivial, and they are offsetting.

The proportions using for the months of January, 1960 through September, 1965 (our interviews began in the following month) are depicted in Figure 2. This gives the proportion of women, born since July 1, 1920 and first married by the month concerned, who reported that they used the pill in that month. The series shows uninterrupted increase at an increasing rate. Words are scarcely necessary to convey the demographic and social interest of this time series.

We have also prepared separate time series of the oral calendar for women first married since the pill was licensed for contraceptive prescription (1960) and for women first married before that time. The average proportions who were using in each month 1961-65 are shown in Table 2. It is evident that use is much more common among recently married wives than among those married a longer time but that use is increasing rapidly in both marital duration categories.

TABLE 2 Per Cent Using Oral Contraception, by Marital Duration, 1961–65

Year	1961	1962	1963	1964	1965
Duration 0–4	3.9	5.5	10.9	15.1	25.6
Duration 5+	0.7	1.7	3.7	7.3	11.1

Table 3 provides a more detailed breakdown of proportions using oral contraceptives at time of interview in late 1965. Had Table 3 alone been considered, it might have led to the inference that women were using the pill early in their marriage and then abandoning it. But on the basis of Figure 2 and Table 2 it is apparent that what we are observing is the growing probability of pill adoption by the more recent cohorts of married couples.

FIGURE 2 Per Cent of Married Women (Husband Present), Born Since Mid-1920, Currently Using Oral Contraceptives, United States, January, 1960–September, 1965

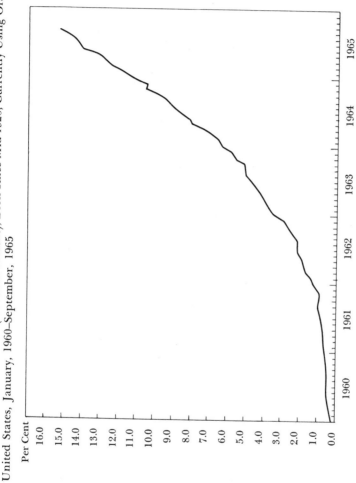

TABLE 3   Per Cent Using Oral Contraception, by Marital Duration, 1965

Duration	0–4	5–9	10–14	15–19	20–24	25+
Per cent using	28.0	22.8	13.4	8.6	5.2	3.7

The strong negative relationship of pill use to marital duration carries the implication of bias in the time series shown in Figure 2. The more recent the year for which proportions are reported, the higher the distribution of women by marital duration. (The women who were married by 1960 were some five years and eight months older by September, 1965.) Had the duration distribution been the same in 1965 as it was in 1960, the proportion currently using would have been 18 per cent rather than 15 per cent. To take this circumstance into account, the duration distribution for each year was estimated, the overall rate for each year adjusted on the basis of the duration-specific proportions shown in Table 3, and new proportions calculated uniformly for marital durations 0-19. The upper duration limit was set because little fertility occurs subsequent to the twentieth year of marriage. The results are shown in Table 4. As expected, Table 4 shows even greater acceleration in use of the pill than Table 2.

TABLE 4   Estimated Per Cent Using, October, 1965 and Years Centered on October, 1960–64, Durations 0–19

Year	1960	1961	1962	1963	1964	1965
Per cent using	0.5	1.1	2.7	6.3	10.9	17.9

V.   THE RELATIONSHIP BETWEEN RISE IN PILL USE AND DECLINE IN FERTILITY

The principal purpose of this paper, and the immediate reason for introducing here the data from the oral calendar (which are to be analyzed subsequently in much more detail) is to determine what relationship may exist between the rise in pill use, on the one hand, and the decline in fertility, on the other.

We have obtained the data necessary for this appraisal in the following way. The fertility rates discussed in Section I are a joint consequence of the fertility of married women, husband present (to which our data on use of the pill apply), and of the proportion of all women in that marital category. We can obtain proportions married, husband present, for 1960 and 1965 from *Current Population Reports,* series P-20, No. 144 (November 10, 1965) for age groups 14-17, 18-19, 20-24, 25-29, 30-34, and 35-44. For the small amount of use of the pill in 1960 we have assumed the same pattern by age as in 1965. It is also assumed that all use reported occurred subsequent to first marriage, and that all fertility reported occurred to women who were married, husband present.

For each of five age groups we have estimated marital fertility rates for 1960 and 1965 by dividing each age-specific fertility rate by the corresponding proportion of women married, husband present. Table 5 shows the per cent decline in marital fertility, 1960-65, and the increase in the proportion of married women using the pill (with a nine-month lead). Examination of the two proportions for each individual age group makes it apparent that the age pattern of decline is quite unlike the age pattern of pill adoption.

TABLE 5   Changes in Marital Fertility and in Pill Use, 1960–65

Age group	Per cent decline in marital fertility	Increase in per cent using pill
14–19	8	17
20–24	20	19
25–29	17	14
30–34	15	8
35–44	18	4
14–44	19	10

The same kind of conclusion emerges from a study of the decline in total fertility year by year and the rise in the proportion using (among durations 0-19), again with a nine-month lead. We see in Table 6 that the decline in total fertility was well in advance of the increase in pill use. (It should be remembered that total fertility also reflects changes in the proportion of women married, husband present.)

181

TABLE 6   Year-by-Year Changes in Total Fertility and in Pill Use, 1960–65

Interval	Per cent decline in total fertility	Increase in per cent using pill
1960–61	1.0	0.3
1961–62	4.0	0.5
1962–63	4.2	1.7
1963–64	4.0	3.6
1964–65	8.4	4.6

A third test seems appropriate. We can examine the per cent decline in the total fertility rate, first order, and the rise in the proportion using, marital duration 0-4. In the period between 1960 and 1965 the first order fertility rate dropped by 17.8 per cent, while the proportion of marital duration 0-4 using the pill (with a lead of nine months ahead of calendar 1965) was 17.7 per cent. This looks like a much more promising comparison. But when we examine the pattern of change through time we find the results shown in Table 7. In short, the similarity noted for 1960-65 is evidently a coincidence, because the annual patterns are quite different. Furthermore, the proportion of women married, husband present, ages 18-24, dropped by 6 per cent between March, 1960 and March, 1965; this drop is reflected in the decline of T.F.R.(I).

TABLE 7   Year-by-Year Changes in First Order Fertility and in Pill Use, Duration 0–4, 1960–65

Interval	Per cent decline in T.F.R. (I)	Rise in per cent using, duration 0–4
1960–61	2.2	1.1
1961–62	4.7	1.6
1962–63	3.0	3.6
1963–64	0.7	4.7
1964–65	8.5	6.0

There are many further questions which must be asked before a clear opinion on the relationship between pill use and fertility decline is achieved. It is our intention to attempt to establish a clear link, for the couples in our study, between their contraceptive behavior and their reproduction, rather

182

than rely on such macroanalytic comparisons as those presented here. In advance of that necessary analysis, it does seem pertinent to note that the oral contraceptive is only one of a battery of procedures which have been employed successfully over a long time, that in late 1965 the majority of women were still employing other contraceptive procedures, and that the use of the pill was very recent. Nevertheless, the acceleration in fertility decline between 1964 and 1965 and the simultaneous acceleration in the adoption of oral contraception is unlikely to be merely a coincidence.

Given the circumstances, one question to which we can never derive a satisfactory answer is: What would the pill users have been using if they hadn't been using the pill? Data from our other paper at this conference suggest that pill use is more likely than not to be a replacement for the condom or the diaphragm, both highly effective contraceptives. It is our hunch that what has been happening to fertility in the 1960's would have happened in direction, if not in degree, even if the oral contraceptive had not appeared on the scene, although the tempo of decline most recently can probably be attributed in part to the availability of this highly efficient and apparently highly acceptable method of fertility regulation.

ANNA L. SOUTHAM

10. BIOLOGICAL DISCOVERIES AND FAMILY PLANNING

The medical literature of ancient times describes numerous methods for the diagnosis and treatment of sterility as well as for the prevention of pregnancy and indicates a longstanding human concern with these problems. Most methods reflect a mystic rather than a rational approach, but the fact that many current methods of contraception are merely refinements of those known in antiquity indicates the startling newness of adequate scientific effort in this area.

THE BIOLOGY OF REPRODUCTION

There are five principal levels concerned with normal fertility. Normal function at each level is dependent on normal function at each preceding level. However, the chain of events is not simple, because of complex interlinkages; a broken link may disturb all preceding as well as subsequent levels.

1. The central nervous system coordinates all humoral and sensory stimuli and releases appropriate chemical messages which control the anterior pituitary gland.

185

2. The anterior pituitary gland, in response to directions from the central nervous system, produces and releases stimulating hormones, the gonadotrophins which act on the ovaries and testes, and "feeds back" the information that it has done so to the hypothalamic area of the central nervous system.

3. The gonads (ovaries and testes) respond to gonadotrophins in a dual fashion by (a) the maturation of ova and production of sperm and (b) the synthesis and release of various sex steroid hormones. The steroid hormones are among the major humoral stimuli which influence the central nervous system and may have a direct effect on the pituitary gland in addition to their effect on the accessory organs of reproduction and on sexual behavior. These first three levels are completely interdependent, and failure at any one level disrupts the other two.

4. The accessory organs of reproduction (the oviducts, uterus, and vagina in the female; the duct system, seminal fluid producing glands, and the penis in the male) respond to steroid hormones by providing a suitable environment for survival and transport of ova and sperm from the gonads to the site of fertilization within the oviduct, for nourishment and transfer of the fertilized ovum to the uterus, and for implantation and growth of the embryo. The cyclic variation in estrogen and progesterone in the female are responsible for changes in uterine and tubal motility, for changes in genital tract secretions, and numerous other factors which favor gestation.

5. Normal sexual behavior is in part dependent on the effect of sex steroids on the genital tract and on central nervous stimuli. In humans and other species of primates, sexual receptivity is not limited to the period of maximum fertility, as it is in lower mammals, and the frequency of timing of coitus are important factors in fertility.

FERTILITY REGULATION

Sterility may be cured or temporary infertility induced by manipulation of several of the above levels.

1. *Central Nervous System*: Specific areas which control the reproductive process have been identified within the central nervous system, and the chemical composition of the controlling substances may soon be known. It is quite possible that once isolated and identified these hypothalamic releasing and inhibiting factors may be used to produce or regulate ovulation, or to suppress it.

Considerable evidence suggests that the hormonal agents currently in use for suppression of ovulation may exert their primary action at the level of the hypothalamus and that other changes in the reproductive sequence are secondary. A great number of compounds which suppress ovulation are available. They consist, in general, of orally active estrogens and progestins taken either in sequence or in combination. The estrogen component is important for its ovulation inhibiting properties and is needed to prime the endometrium to produce regular uterine bleeding. The progestins alone, in adequate doses, may inhibit ovulation, but in most of the currently available tablets the estrogen component is important. Long-acting compounds, given by injection, are in the process of development. It is quite possible that an injection every six to 12 months will prove as effective as the daily administration of the current pills.

2. *Anterior Pituitary Gland*: Gonadotrophins have been extracted from human pituitary glands and from the urine of postmenopausal and pregnant women. These substances are extremely potent and will produce ovulation and pregnancy in certain infertile women but are not as yet approved for general use.

Contraceptive agents which act primarily at the level of the anterior pituitary gland are not yet available although a number of compounds which may act as antigonadotrophins have been investigated. Immunological neutralization of gonadotrophins with resultant suppression of ovulation or spermatogenesis has been achieved in laboratory animals.

3. *Gonads*: There is no indication that infertility due to complete ovarian or testicular failure can be corrected.

In some women, infertile because of lack of ovulation, a simple substance taken by mouth for a few days produces ovulation. This compound (clomiphene citrate) is being tested for its ability to regulate ovulation and thus produce a predictable fertile time, and, while still in the clinical testing stage, it may become a useful adjunct to the regulation of fertility in the future. It is uncertain as yet whether this drug works at the level of the central nervous system or at the ovarian level, but it facilitates release of endogenous gonadotrophins.

Evidence for and against a direct effect of ovulation suppressing drugs on the ovary has been presented and immunological suppression of ovarian function has been reported. Heat and a number of chemical agents appear to inhibit sperm production at the testicular level without interfering with testicular hormone production, and immunological aspermatogenesis has been produced in men as well as in experimental animals. Substances which appear to produce a transient decrease in the progesterone production necessary for implantation are being subjected to limited clinical trials.

4. *Accessory Organs of Reproduction*: Little is known about the factors which govern ovum and sperm transport, fertilization, and implantation in humans, and the work done in small laboratory animals cannot be considered applicable. A number of workers are studying these problems in sub-human primates in which the reproductive physiology more closely resembles that of women. Contraceptives which act only at the tubal or uterine level seem more desirable medically than those affecting higher centers.

The use of intra-uterine foreign bodies to decrease fertility or to treat infertility is an ancient technique. For centuries, Arabian and Turkish camel owners have used intra-uterine contraception to prevent pregnancy in their saddle animals. Their technique was simple. A small stone (pessary) was inserted into the uterus through a hollow tube. The nineteenth-century medical literature on intra-uterine pessaries is voluminous, but it has been only in the last five years that this method has been scientifically evaluated and its usefulness defined. The mechanism by which intra-uterine devices (IUD) prevent pregnancy varies from species to species and is still under investigation. Under certain experimental conditions, they appear to hasten tubal transport of unfertilized ova in subhuman primates. Although the exact mechanism in women is not yet clearly defined, the collected evidence indicates that intra-uterine contraception exerts its effect on either tubal or uterine factors before implantation. The devices do not interfere with sperm migration. Suggestions that they act by producing abortion or uterine infection have been discredited. Intra-uterine contraception decreases tubal as well as intra-uterine implantation, suggesting rapid ovum transport.

The usual combinations of synthetic estrogens and progestins which inhibit ovulation have a direct effect on endometrial development and cervical mucus consistency which may, perhaps incidentally, contribute to contraceptive effectiveness. However, some progestational agents alone, by producing minor alterations in physiology, may be highly effective contraceptive agents when given in amounts too small to inhibit ovulation. Clinical trials now under way suggest that the estrogen effect on cervical mucus may be eliminated, thus providing a barrier to sperm migration, or that the estrogen priming necessary for endometrial secretory response to progesterone may be altered. Such a method theoretically would not cause a physiological imbalance or produce side effects and would be an ideal method from the medical viewpoint. It is quite possible that reservoirs within the body or food supplements could provide long-term yet readily reversible protection.

Other preliminary work suggests that rather large doses of synthetic estrogens administered to rhesus monkeys and to women during the first few days following ovulation may prevent pregnancy, perhaps through an effect on tubal transport of the ovum.

5. *Sexual Behavior:* This complex subject will be considered only as it relates to fertility. Couples often seek to increase or decrease fertility by means of timed sexual intercourse. Unfortunately there is no accurate simple method for the determination of either the fertile or the infertile period. In most experimental animals, the functional survival time of spermatozoa does not exceed 48 hours, and the ovum must be promptly fertilized if it is to develop normally. Fer-

189

tilization occurring more than eight hours after ovulation results in a high percentage of abnormal embryos which are incapable of surviving. If the same situation pertains in humans, conception is possible for no more than three days during each menstrual cycle. However, there is some evidence that sperm retain their fertilizing capacity for five or six days in the Fallopian tubes of the mare, and conceptions have been reported with controlled insemination in humans done five or six days before the estimated time of ovulation. Much indirect evidence has accumulated suggesting that the most fertile time in women is about 15 days before the next expected menstrual period, or during the 48 hours before the basal body temperature chart reflects the thermogenic effects of progesterone. There is a widespread erroneous belief that the temperature rise marks the most fertile time of a woman's cycle. Many couples, with apparent infertility, have been incorrectly advised to abstain from intercourse before the temperature rise in order to "save" sperm for the supposed moment of ovulation. These infertile couples are unwittingly practicing effective rhythm contraception and conceive promptly when coitus occurs a day or two earlier. The length of time from ovulation to menstruation is relatively constant. Variations in the length of the menstrual cycle are due chiefly to variations in the pre-ovulatory phase—the time required for a follicle to grow to maturity and release an ovum following onset of the preceding menstrual period. Few women have absolutely regular cycles and ovulation cannot yet be predicted far enough in advance of the event to define the onset of the fertile time. The information that ovulation has occurred can be obtained from numerous tests and signs. The simplest and least expensive so far is observation of the basal body temperature pattern.

Periodic abstinence, the use of condoms, *coitus interruptus,* spermicidal agents of various types, and occlusive devices involve modifications of coital technique to prevent sperm from reaching a viable ovum and are very old methods. They differ from previously described methods in that they require planned continence or action at the time of sexual intercourse and demand greater sustained motivation.

SAFETY OF CONTRACEPTIVE METHODS

Ovulation Suppression: Inhibition of the reproductive process at the central nervous system level requires consideration of the effect of consequent changes on all other hormonally influenced structures and function, and these are many. In addition, total body exposure to the inhibiting drugs produces side effects of a systemic nature and imposes contraindications in cases where the changes in metabolism might unfavorably influence the course of an existing disease. The metabolic changes produced by endogenous and exogenous steroids have been considered at two World Health Organization Scientific Group meetings, one in 1965 and one in 1966. The significance of undesired secondary effects of hormonal contraception was considered, and further research on the long-term consequences of current methods was recommended.

Disruption of the reproductive sequence at any level modifies function at all subsequent levels. Lower links in the chain may perhaps be broken with less concern for potentially serious systemic side effects.

Intra-uterine Contraception: The side effects associated with the use of intra-uterine contraceptive devices are chiefly local in nature and contraindications to the use of this method involve only pelvic factors. The insertion of an intra-uterine device is simple but requires skill if serious complications of the method such as infection or uterine perforation are to be avoided.

Antiestrogens: Progestational drugs which act at the level of the accessory organs and do not inhibit ovulation must be administered systemically to reach the accessory organs, and therefore consideration must be given to generalized side effects. These seem to be minimal, however, and on a theoretical basis few would be expected.

Periodic Abstinence: Lack of precision in identification of the fertile period limits the effectiveness of this method and creates anxiety in those for whom reliability is a first consideration. On the basis of findings in experimental animals, embryologists suggest that increased fetal wastage or anomalies might result from delayed fertilization associated

191

with failures of this method; this probably has not been confirmed in humans.

Other Methods: There are essentially no known side effects associated with the use of condoms or of *coitus interruptus*, although these methods may lack acceptance on esthetic grounds in some cultures. The various spermicidal preparations may produce local irritations, but contraindications to their use are few.

Carcinogenesis: Concern exists regarding possible carcinogenic effects of contraceptive agents. The problem of analysis is complicated by lack of information as to the expected incidence of premalignant and malignant changes in the female genital tract in various populations. Many long-term studies are in progress as part of steroid and intra-uterine contraception projects. Preliminary reports from investigators in several countries indicate that neither method increases the risk of genital tract cancer.

EFFECTIVENESS

The effectiveness of contraception is measured by failure rates and expressed as unintended pregnancies per hundred woman years of use. Failure rates reflect the use effectiveness of a method, since no distinction can be made between method failure and patient failure. It is quite possible that theoretical effectiveness is similar for most methods, since low as well as high failure rates have been reported in selected series of carefully supervised acceptors using rhythm, condoms, diaphragms, and spermicidal agents as well as steroid and intra-uterine contraception. However, theoretical effectiveness is a relatively useless measure if the degree of motivation required is unrealistic for the intended users. The use effectiveness of intra-uterine contraception is equal to its theoretical effectiveness, since only initial motivation is needed and reversal requires a positive step—removal of the device. Before the use effectiveness of the combination oral contraceptives differs greatly from its theoretical effectiveness, several tablets must be omitted. The degree to which omission contributes to the higher failure rates of other methods is not known.

ACCEPTABILITY

A general comparison of the acceptability of contraceptive methods is not possible, as this varies among individuals and among nationalities. Reported discontinuing rates of oral contraceptors range from 6 to 74 per cent within the first year of use. Approximately 30 per cent of women in IUD series have discontinued by the end of one year. The number of couples accepting and continuing to use a given method depends on many factors besides free choice of known methods. Not least among these many factors are availability and cost.

It has been estimated that perhaps 15 per cent of currently eligible couples throughout the world are using contraceptive materials of some type. Enough condoms are produced each year throughout the world to supply approximately 12 to 15 million couples (12 to 13 million gross). An estimated eight million women use oral contraception, and approximately five million use spermicidal preparations either with or without diaphragms. More than one million women are already wearing intra-uterine devices, and goals set for national programs may multiply this by many times within the next few years. In some countries *coitus interruptus* is the most widely used method; techniques depending on male initiative or cooperation (as in periodic continence) are more widely used than any other in many countries of the world. This fact may have important implications for the development of new types of contraceptives.

Only ten years have passed since the introduction of oral contraception. This first really new method in more than a century was developed through the rational application of scientific knowledge to a problem, but all of the basic information necessary to make this development a reality had been published at least 15 years before. Intra-uterine devices have been used for centuries, but research to improve and evaluate this method is less than five years old. Known biological facts are now being used to develop new methods, and we can hope that, as new basic discoveries in the field of reproductive biology emerge, applied research can yield even more sophisticated and effective methods of family planning.

DISCUSSION

The following presentations of four authors contain predictions and suggestions in relation to the topics discussed in the papers of Dr. Southam, Mr. Westoff and Mr. Ryder.

In separate discussions of the Ryder and Westoff papers, Raymond Potvin and Michael F. Valente consider the significance of the pill as a contraceptive medium. Father Potvin questions the lower fertility rate and the extent to which the pill is responsible for the decline. Mr. Valente feels the percentage of women using the pill is large considering its newness. He suggests that the pill may be responsible for an increase in the percentage of persons practicing birth control. Both men comment on the effect of contraception on the Church's theological position. Father Potvin asks if it is necessary for theologians to consider human behavior and motivations when discussing relevant issues.

A summary of future contraceptive devices is given by Dr. Gordon Perkin and Thomas P. Carney in their discussions of Dr. Southam's paper, "Biological Discoveries and Family Planning." Dr. Perkin predicts the approximate order in which the newer fertility controls will become available. Mr. Carney suggests consequent future research and discusses some problems that may arise as a result of the new methods. He asks researchers to concentrate on the practical application of their knowledge.*

*Drs. William Masters and Virginia Johnson of the Washington University Medical School also spoke at this time, reporting on their laboratory work concerning the change of sex organs and clinical correction of the malfunctioning of sex organs. In the course of their remarks, reasons for "rhythm failures," based on their laboratory findings, were presented. Since such works are still in the process of being analyzed, Drs. Masters and Johnson preferred that their reports be omitted from the Conference proceedings (Ed.).

194

POTVIN: I should like to draw some implications from the Westoff and Ryder papers. It is important to keep in mind that lower period fertility rates do not necessarily mean that eventual family size is being reduced or that fewer children are being or will be born. This can be seen in the Ryder paper, especially in the creative technique of controlling for changes in time patterns of childbearing. In effect, a reduction in birth rates can be simply or partly a postponement of children. So the recent drop in period rates does not mean that the American people are aware of a population problem or that we do not have anything to worry about. Therefore, the question of motivation for responsible family planning is still an important one and I do not think there is any reason for complacency in the fact of presently declining birth or fertility rates. This is one point worth discussing.

The second point I wish to make on the Ryder paper is that the pattern of percentage decline in fertility and the percentage use of the pill are not alike. It is then suggested that the decline may be due to other factors than the pill. I think this is true, but, as the authors have pointed out, it is the young persons who are adopting the pill more than other groups. Their conclusion that "the acceleration in fertility decline between 1964 and 1965 and the simultaneous acceleration in the adoption of oral contraception is unlikely to be merely a coincidence," needs explanation. It may be that younger persons are postponing or limiting births which they may not have done otherwise if it were not for the pill. This is especially crucial, since in another part of their paper they mention that there has been a postponement of first births. To what extent is this postponement due to the pill? Previous studies have shown that a lower proportion of younger women, married less than five years, have used contraception than in other age groups. To what extent was this lower proportion due to problems with method? It may be that the pill is making a psychological difference for these younger couples in that the act of intercourse and the act of contraception are clearly separate. This may be part of the explanation for the postponement of first births for the most recent cohort. It would be interesting to check this out.

About the Westoff paper, I should like to say that the authors

195

have pointed out difficulties in clearly distinguishing between users of the pill for contraceptive motives and for medical reasons. They did not, however, specify the problem. As I see it, the intent on the part of Catholics to regularize the cycle can be answered or interpreted as contraceptive intent because this is why they want to regularize the cycle. But it also can be answered or interpreted as a medical reason, namely that their cycle is not normal and, hence, they are using medical means to regularize it. It is possible, therefore, that because of this confusion the nonconformers to traditional Catholic doctrine may be inflated. This should be kept in mind while interpreting the statistics. I believe from talking to Westoff that the authors can solve this problem eventually from some of the other data they have but have not analyzed.

In spite of this issue, I believe it fair to say that regularly practicing Catholics are increasingly using methods that have not been officially approved by their Church. But, for the theologian, how meaningful is the category "methods ever used"? It lumps persons who have used a method once with others who have used it regularly for years. Nonconformity, therefore, means entirely different forms of behavior. Obviously, the authors have used this category of "methods ever used" for comparative purposes, but I believe future analysis should distinguish between a rare user and a consistent one, because theologically they are entirely different problems.

The reason I bring this up is that the theological position has been advanced by some authors that the theologian should take into account human behavior; not in the sense that human behavior changes theological positions, but that when the Christian conscience is witnessing, when you see Christians attempting to live according to their principles yet nonetheless violating some official doctrine, this is an occasion for theologians to reevaluate their assumptions and possibly change their position. For example, at one time most theologians taught that having intercourse with one's wife when she was pregnant was sinful, but many conscientious Christians could not accept the doctrine and eventually the theology changed. I do not know the cause of the change, but there was an empirical association at least. Some of these data in the Westoff paper, therefore, may be relevant for theologians, because we do know that persons who are more religious are also in that process of getting further away from the traditional doctrine. We should clarify for theologians exactly what is going on. Whether religious Catholics use a nonapproved method one week or 10 years does make a difference.

VALENTE: I found it very interesting to learn from the papers of Ryder and Westoff that in late 1965 a considerable number of married women were using the oral contraceptive. As the paper points out, "the majority of women were still employing other contraceptive procedures"; nevertheless, those using the pill represent a very significant number, particularly when one considers the comparative newness of the method. I am surprised not that the percentage is small but that it is so large. Moreover, as Ryder and Westoff point out, this percentage has been increasing. I would be very interested in knowing whether or not it will continue to do so and why or why not. Perhaps a future study will provide us with this data.

I fully agree that we can never satisfactorily answer the question which Ryder and Westoff pose, namely, "What would the pill users have been using if they hadn't been using the pill?" Nevertheless, I wonder if one might reasonably claim that pill users would have been using a less effective and, particularly, a less attractive method. I think that Ryder and Westoff suggest that other less desirable methods would be used. They tell us that "the pill has been adopted primarily by couples who would otherwise have used, or were formerly using, the diaphragm, the condom, or the rhythm method." In the context of the United States of the 1960's, I do not think there is widespread absolute determination to reduce one's fertility at any cost and means. Rather, I think there is a widespread orientation toward conception control within the framework of the small-family system. This seems significant. All of us know of a child who was an accident, who arrived ahead of schedule or who was not intended at all. This does not bespeak absolute determination but suggests a percentage of human error within a general contraceptive setting. If the pill significantly reduces this percentage of error, it seems that it has had and could continue to have an important effect on family planning. Clearly, it is much more attractive to some groups than the condom, diaphragm, or rhythm method

197

because of its simplicity, method, and particularly its physical absence at the time of intercourse. This latter element removes the stark consciousness of a direct interference and substitutes an action similar to taking an aspirin.

The popularity of the pill brings me to my next consideration. Ryder and Westoff tell us that for both Catholic and non-Catholic there has been a trend toward increased use of the oral contraceptive. They also note this trend was observed between 1955 and 1960.

This poses a serious ethical question for Roman Catholics, a question of which we are all acutely aware and of which theologians have been aware for a long time. Yet, no answer is forthcoming, apparently because doubt does exist in the Roman Catholic Church on the subject of contraception, despite Pope Paul's assertion [October, 1966] to the contrary. The effect of the Pope's manner of response to this climate of doubt has produced a situation in which there is a changing relation to authority. This means that the Catholic behavior pattern is not as easily predictable as it may have been at one time.

On the one hand, there is clearly a freer use of contraceptive devices in general and the pill in particular. Catholic husbands and wives who are not justifying this use through a process of theological ratiocination, really do not have to. Many confessors regularly advise penitents to follow their conscience in deciding the means of planning. Those with whom I am acquainted have been doing so for quite a few years.

On the other hand, some couples who feel they must practice birth control cannot justify their action. As a result, some lose interest in the Mass, where they are excluded from reception of the sacraments and the life of God and his Church. Seeing themselves cut off spiritually, they are unwilling to live a lie and thus cut themselves off physically.

This situation is clearly unjust and leads the theologian to pose yet another important ethical question: Since 1964, what is the ethical content of the actions of the Pope, who refuses to acknowledge the existence of doubt in the Church, vis-à-vis the Birth Control Commission, which came out of the deliberations of the bishops in assembly at Vatican II together with the theologians?[1]

[1] These remarks made by Mr. Valente were pertinent at the time the Conference was held in December, 1966 (Ed.).

Finally, the pill introduces the possibility of one-sided decision making within the family and thus poses ethical questions much like those suggested by the debates over "cooperation," which was a point of intense theological interest for several hundred years.

PERKIN: It is my hope that the social scientists, the demographers, and the theologians present will consider the challenge of initiating prospective studies and formulating positions on the moral and theological questions which the new methods raise, while the methods are being clinically evaluated. I would like to present several of the newer contraceptive developments in the approximate order in which they are likely to become available in the United States and throughout the world.

Initially, I would like to consider an existing method, the intra-uterine device. As the acceptance and the widespread use of this method increase, we are beginning to see encouraging signs of specialized medical and engineering talent directed towards the development of new and improved devices. While the action mechanism of the device in humans has still to be conclusively proven, there is no evidence to contradict Dr. Mastroiannis' findings that in superovulated artificially inseminated monkeys the device acts by speeding passage of the egg from the ovary to the uterus so that it arrives ahead of schedule and is probably "unfertilizable." None of the ova that he has recovered to date have been fertilized.

Oral contraceptives: There are presently 12 products marketed by seven companies in the United States. The presentation by Westoff and Ryder demonstrated the high acceptance and the exceptional degree to which this method is used throughout the country. Because of the popularity of "the pill" and because of the potential commercial market, we are witnessing a highly competitive race among manufacturers who want to capture or increase their share of the market. In the immediate future (the Food and Drug Administration willing), we are likely to see a continued proliferation of closely related competing compounds, such as more sequential preparations and more low dose compounds. We will also begin to have available modifications in dosage schedule; for example, a 21-tablet monthly regimen rather than the current 20. The patient would be instructed to take the medication three weeks out of four, simplifying the instruction that is currently necessary with the present dosage schedule.

We will also begin to see continuous therapy where placebos are administered during the period of withdrawal bleeding or where very low doses of estrogen are given during this period. This will permit the patient taking a pill every day to avoid the necessity of counting or of adhering to a strict schedule involving dates.

Oral products, then, will continue to compete on the claims of lower dose, reduced side effects, more physiological action, improved packaging, or simpler schedule of administration.

One of the more significant modifications in the oral control of conception (through hormones) that is likely to appear in the near future is the injectable steroid. Currently at least two companies are conducting large-scale clinical evaluations of injectable compounds which provide protection over periods of one, three, or as long as six months following a single injection. Some problems of irregular bleeding during the treatment and varying periods of amenorrhea (absence of menses) following discontinuation of the therapy may limit their widespread acceptance.

The injectable approach however appears to be sufficiently popular with women in the study groups to predict a significant future role for this method. Rather than requiring a single decision on the part of the woman as with the IUD, or repetitive, coitally connected decisions as with the traditional methods of birth control, the injectable approach requires relatively infrequent, yet regular visits to medical personnel for administration of the compound. Is it possible for sociologists to predict which women are likely to accept and prefer this method and which ones will use it consistently as the method of controlling their family size?

Perhaps, the most interesting development on the horizon and one that may become a reality in the very near future is the use of microdose oral contraceptives. To be consistent with the theme that has run through this conference, I think we should then refer to the existing contraceptive compounds as macrodoses and to the new ones as microdoses.

It has been shown that the very small doses, .2 and .4 milligrams, of several of the presently used progestational agents are also effective in preventing pregnancy. The significant difference ap-

200

pears to be the mechanism of action. These compounds are administered daily in very small doses. Normal menstruation occurs. The normal menstrual cycle is not generally affected, and ovulation is not inhibited in the majority of cases. The question is how do these compounds work. We are still not sure, but among the possibilities, they may alter tubal transport time, alter cervical mucus to render it hostile to sperm, or change endometrial receptivity so that implantation is prevented.

There are certainly some medical advantages to these microdose compounds; they do not suppress the pituitary gland, yet they provide effective local action through systemic medication. What theological questions are raised by a drug whose mechanism of action (inhibition of ovulation) at one dosage level has received widespread use and growing theological acceptance, when it is shown that the same drug is equally effective in preventing pregnancy at a much lower dosage level but by a different mechanism of action?

There are several interesting possible applications of these microdose progestational compounds. The first one most likely to become available is the daily pill. The advantages in this case are that each tablet would be identical, packaging would be simplified; a year's supply of 365 tablets could be placed in a single bottle. The patient is instructed to take a pill every day. Also, with the reduced content of progestational compound, the cost of the drug becomes much less significant, thus increasing the possibility of this method being widely used, particularly in developing countries.

A second possible way in which the microdose concept may be utilized is to combine it with essential amino acids in a wafer or biscuit form to provide women their nutritional status and health while protecting them from further pregnancy. (This was originally suggested as somewhat of a jest but is now being researched.) In many developing countries if the woman is unable to nurse her baby because of health reasons or debility, the infant will die from a lack of protein. The opportunity to improve a mother's nutritional status and to protect her from a subsequent pregnancy would decrease both infant and maternal mortality and morbidity.

The third and most intriguing but presently the least conceiv-

201

able utilization of the microdose concept is its application in a depot form. There are studies today in which chlormadinone, one of the compounds being used, has been placed in a silastic pellet. This is a synthetic, inert rubber material which can be embedded under the skin. The active compound is "leached out" or released slowly over a prolonged period of time. This approach has been shown to be successful in rodents. It is presently being tested in primates, and there is a great deal of optimism over the possible advantages of this particular application. The pellet, placed in the patient's arm at or shortly after the time of delivery, would provide sustained protection with only a single decision on the part of the patient. The patient could return to have the pellet removed at any time or she might be given a very small dose of estrogen at a critical time during the cycle to counteract the effect of the embedded drug and permit pregnancy to occur.

The post-coital pill has received considerable attention from the lay press in the past few months. Dr. Chang at Worchester has shown that doses of selected progestins given at critical times prior to ovulation and doses of estrogens given at critical times following ovulation are successful in reducing the number of implantation sites in rodents. Dr. Morris at Yale has shown that the post-coital administration of synthetic antiestrogen or high doses of synthetic estrogens given post-coitally will prevent implantation in primates. These compounds may act by reducing tubal transport time or by subtly altering the endometrium so that implantation does not occur. Although such a method is unlikely to become available in the United States for a number of years, it is quite possible that present testing in a number of Eastern European and Asian countries may lead to the availability and widespread use of such a method.

There are several compounds which increase fertility. The best known are pergenol and clomiphene. I think it is quite likely that either or both of these agents will soon become available to physicians. What will be the official position of the Church on the administration of chemical compounds to barren women which artificially produce ovulation resulting in pregnancy?

Finally, reports are continually being published on animal studies linking delayed fertilization to significantly increased rates of spontaneous abortion and abnormal pregnancy. A recent medical report attributed the cause of tubal pregnancies to delayed fertilization. The possibility exists, therefore, that the rhythm method, which frequently involves delayed fertilization or fertilization of a so-called "old ovum," is not without some risk.

In summary, it is encouraging to note the growing scientific attention devoted to the development of new approaches to fertility control. There also appears to be growing support for and interest in methods which require a positive action to have a further pregnancy rather than a continuing series of negative actions to keep from becoming pregnant. With the intra-uterine device and the long-acting hormone implants, women must take some action to become pregnant rather than continuing to do something to prevent pregnancy. Increasing attention is also being focused on the events between ovulation and implantation with the search for compounds which will successfully intervene at the local level. Agents affecting tubal motility, ovum transport and implantation are likely to represent the next generation of contraceptive methods. There appears to be a unique opportunity for the disciplines represented at this meeting to join with the clinical-medical researcher and begin considering the many questions which will require answers in the coming years.

CARNEY: Dr. Southam's paper is my only real area of competence. There is nothing in her paper that bears discussion or disagreement, but I do think that Dr. Southam missed an opportunity to discuss some of the more promising future research. Someone used to describe one of the thermodynamics laws as not being able to push on something that is moving away faster than you are. Sometimes when we consider these problems, we consider them as they are today, not as they might be tomorrow.

Commenting on Dr. Perkin's discussion, I think the things about which he talked have almost materialized; the 28- and 21-day pills are already on sale in other countries around the world. The long-term contraceptive, I think, could be made available almost any time anyone wanted it. It will be some time before it is available in this country, because of our food and drug regulations.

In considering use for contraceptives, we should think of the objective and decide if it is only demographic. Are we interested

203

only in decreasing population or are we interested also in the humanistic reaction? In other words, I would feel more comfortable about rendering contraceptives to reduce population if I could say that 95 or 97 per cent were effective. I do not think you can feel that comfortable when you are talking to one woman and telling her that this material assures that she will not have a baby. We have to consider this in deciding what will be available in the future.

Let me tell you about some of today's research. This work is being done with animals. Some of it has been in a clinic. Scientists doing research in any kind of population control are interested in both the ovum and the sperm. A great deal of work has been done on the sperm. There are many women today who have born babies as a result of artificial insemination from material that has been stored in sperm banks.

I would like to mention some issues with which sociologists and theologians may have to deal if the use of artificial insemination becomes more widespread. Let us picture a savings bank for a man. He will deposit sperm in the bank, which he can withdraw on demand. In view of the discussion about mutual agreement, I do not know whether it should be a joint account. I do not know whether a woman should be allowed to withdraw it. This is a practical problem. If artificial insemination becomes a socially acceptable practice, it opens up all kinds of possibilities.

One of the objections to total sterilization has been that this is an irrevocable decision. Once either the man or the woman is sterilized, the couple can not have children. However, the possibility of sperm banks eliminates to some degree that kind of objection. A man at the time of his marriage could deposit sperm that would be available for the rest of his life. He could be sterilized and artificial insemination could be used so the couple could have children. This is a totally practical thing.

There is much work being done on what might be called the invetral fertilization of ova. Ova and sperm can be collected and the ova can be literally fertilized in a test tube. This has been done, and considerable work is going on in Italy, France, and particularly Japan. Also, attempts are actually being made at the clinical level to transplant a fertilized ovum to a woman's uterus. We have sufficient knowledge to control what is required for the fertilized ovum to successfully lodge on the uterine wall. All factors involved are known and can be controlled by chemicals. This is not only a clinical experiment. There is a material on the market from our laboratories that controls ovulation of animals, making artificial insemination possible. Some of the materials stimulate superovulation. A cow, for example, given these hormones, may produce a hundred ova. The ova can be removed from the cow. Sperm can be collected from a bull and all of these ova can be fertilized invetrally. The ova can then be transferred to other cows and normal calves will be born. This means that you can take one thoroughbred cow, one thoroughbred bull and get a hundred thoroughbred calves from scrub cows. This is actually being done.

Another rather dramatic experiment which received a lot of publicity has been the isolation of an ovum from a yew, fertilization of that ovum invetrally, the transference of the fertilized ovum to the uterus of a rabbit, the transportation of that rabbit to another country, isolation of the embryo from the rabbit, transplantation of the embryo into another yew, and the birth of a normal lamb. These things could be done for human beings.

Dr. Perkin mentioned the stimulation of ovulation. Again, this is practical and is being done. He mentioned two compounds which are being used, clomiphene and pergenol. Pergenol, I think, has a broader use, but presently it is not generally as controllable. It has been used somewhat recklessly. You have probably seen the publicity on some of the multiple births resulting from this, such as the sextuplets who later died. There was another case where there were 12 embryos present in a woman. From work that is being carried on in Israel and England, I believe that the compounds are controllable, but the process involves an examination almost every day and a daily titration of the woman to stimulate only one ovum.

Stanford University has quite a program dealing with this type of continuation of the invetral kind of growth. They are recovering very small embryos which are spontaneously ejected and are trying to construct an artificial uterus. Presently, they have a pressure chamber in which they add oxygen and are able to keep some of these extremely small and new ebryos living for some days.

205

With the possibility of the transplantation of a fertilized ovum into a human being, a few wild suggestions have been made as to the consequences. They are wild, though, only when you think of them in the abstract. As you know, a woman suffering from an Rh problem is placed at a more critical stage. According to the number of children she has, the Rh antibodies build up and she has trouble with subsequent children. There is now a table of women who will volunteer as subjects for the transplantation of a fertilized egg from the uterus of a woman who anticipates an Rh problem. The volunteer woman would carry the fertilized egg to term, but whose baby would it be?

In the not too distant future, it will be possible to control the sex of a human being; this again is being done in animals. We are finding out more and more about the differences in properties between male and female sperm. The difference between an X and Y chromosome is more than that. It is physical difference. In some animals, the male and female sperm can be separated by physical methods. If you could justify the use of artificial insemination, you could inseminate either the male or the female sperm and assure the sex of the offspring.

Dr. Perkin also mentioned long-acting contraceptive materials. One which is now in use was just put into a long-acting form. The other material will be released in very small quantities. I am reserving judgment both on the mechanism of action and the utility of those materials. One theory of the action of compounds claims that progestins simply increase the amount of cervical mucus, which then acts as a physical barrier. In all the work that I have seen, the sperm that is embedded in this mucus can be recovered as a viable, motile sperm. The mucus does not kill the sperm. With the hundreds of millions of sperm in the uterus mucus, it seems that some of them might get through the physical barrier. I do not think there has been enough work done to guarantee 100 per cent effectiveness. Obviously, these things could be used for population controls for demographic purposes.

Before I came here, I read a paper from Cambridge not only discussing contraception but stimulation of sex by means of perfumes. It was a rather dramatic kind of article published in a newspaper which quoted a paper of which I had a pre-publication copy. It pointed out some experiments with certain animals that have a contraceptive perfume for other animals. In certain species of mice, if a male is brought into contact with a female who has had copulation with a normal father, there will be no births from that female. It was discovered that it is a scent emanated from the second breed of mice which causes this contraception. The article was published because a statistician had looked at the times of conception and discovered that the lowest rate was immediately after Christmas. He claimed that this was a result of so much perfume being given at Christmas time, which overcame the natural sex perfume attractant. This has about the same validating statistics as the fact that burlesque shows cause persons to become bald-headed since all men in the front row are bald-headed.

Parthenogenesis, the fertilization of an ovum without sperm, is something to think of as practical. It sounds impossible, but for some of the lower animals it has worked. You can get the fertilized ovum of rabbits, for example, and have rabbits without a father.

The final consideration in the ultimate of scientific progress is syntheses of organisms. This also is past speculation. Living organisms have been synthesized in two ways: either by starting with a degraded virus and putting the dead chemicals together again, or by literally synthesizing a living human organism, as the University of Chicago did. If you have a living organism, have knowledge of enzyme, amino acid, and protein involvements, it is possible to take small incomes of change and think about synthesizing a part of a human being, a sperm or an egg for example.

These are some of the things I think of as a scientist, when I think of the overall involvement of sociologists, theologians, demographers, and scientists discussing sociological problems as they involve population. I wish I could say that this is the extent of my involvement, that here are a dozen ways for preventing conception and here are a couple of ways for increasing conception. Unfortunately, I have not been able to do that. It seems that the popular conception of the scientist is somebody who should look at his data coldly and objectively and turn it over to somebody else for use. But, I believe, the time for that kind of activity is past. I think that certainly the scientist should look at his data objectively, but once a decision has been reached he should use whatever emotion, passion, or responsibility he can muster to make his ideas clear and to educate persons who do not recognize the significance of these results.

I might mention how I became involved in the population problem. I have been doing medical research for a long time. In fact, I started almost at the time of the revolution of medical research, when sulfa drugs and antibiotics were being discovered. Before that time there was no way to control even infectious diseases, no way to save children. Since then, I have seen the development of antibiotics in my own laboratory and the records of the lives they have saved. I have seen the materials that I have developed to relieve pain. I thought that the world was a pretty wonderful place in which to live and I was contributing to it.

In working with a great research organization, it is obvious that you cannot tell them to think only in certain narrow fields. Other things arose and we became interested in agricultural research. And, again from my laboratories, I saw materials developed that would increase the feed efficiency of animals, thus increasing the amount of meat. I saw materials that could be put in cotton and corn fields which would practically eliminate tilling, and again I thought I was making quite a contribution.

Then it was time to tie everything together. Here we were relieving human suffering and hunger, and I found to my amazement that it was much easier to think of finding remedies for all the diseases than to think of feeding all the persons in the world. Maybe this is because you can consider medicine almost as a static kind of problem. If you find a polio vaccine, it does not make much difference whether the incidence of polio is increasing or not. You simply make twice as big a batch of vaccine and vaccinate more persons. If you discover the incidence of hunger is increasing, you have a different problem. You know what the cure is, but there is nothing you can do about doubling the batch, at least in any recognizable period of time.

In the lifetime of my children there will be four times as many persons living on the earth as there are now, if the birth rate does not increase or if the life span or the death rate does not change. I think this is a sobering thought. Four times as many persons as there are now with no change. But I know that at least one thing will change. I know that the death rate will decrease

208

because I and other persons in my profession are going to make it go down. We cannot hold up the progress of medical research; it would be monstrous to try to solve a problem like that. And so I decided to enter this area.

If I sound impatient, I guess it is because I am a little. When we talk about spending all of our energies trying to make rhythm practical, about waiting for theological decisions from the French, Germans, or the Italians, when we spend valuable political time talking about whether or not someone who has had five children in five years by five different unknown men would be stimulated to promiscuity by the use of contraceptives, when we talk about whether giving information is courage, I think we are sitting on the bank waiting for the river to pass. I am impatient when I think that since we started this conference there are more than 300,000 more persons on the earth than there were then. This is not just 300,000 births but an actual increase of 300,000 in our population. What are we going to do about them? After the alumni conference on population, one of the persons in the audience came up to me and said, "What advice can you give me about my daughter? She has been married for ten years and has eight children. She ovulates twice a month. Her confessor tells her to use rhythm." These are the kinds of problems about which I think we should talk.

During this symposium, we have been talking about the problems in a rather comfortable, almost abstract, way. We have been talking within our little sphere where we have been collecting data. It seems to me that to discuss problems and get intellectual stimulation from them, to enjoy them without discussing the solution to the problem, is just a type of mental masturbation. We receive temporary enjoyment, but we do not do anything to plant a seed that might result in something really practical.

PART FIVE

Family Planning and Economic Development

LYLE SAUNDERS

11. FAMILY PLANNING,
THE WORLDWIDE VIEW

The concept of family planning can be approached in several ways. In the sense of deliberate acts by married or cohabiting couples to prevent or achieve conception or avoid unwanted births after conception has occurred, family planning is as old as history. Himes (see reference list, item 1), and Noonan (2), among others, have traced the existence of contraceptive and abortion knowledge and practice among preliterate peoples and through much of recorded history in both Oriental and Occidental civilizations. As an organized social movement aimed at attaining economic, political, social, or moral ends through control over conception and birth, family planning dates back about a century and a half. In its most recent manifestation, in the form of large-scale efforts by national governments to decrease rates of population growth, family planning is newer than nuclear fission. What is common to all approaches is an attempt to influence the reproductive behavior of individual couples.

Although every *intended* conception and every *wanted* birth are also properly viewed as outcomes of family planning, the term is most commonly used to refer to actions or

213

programs intended to prevent conception or avoid its consequences when it does occur. This is the sense in which it will
be used throughout this paper, unless otherwise indicated.

There is no accurate way of knowing how much family
planning is going on now or went on at any time in the past.
The concept involves both motivation (in the sense of intention) and sexual behavior, and neither has been adequately
studied even for samples of national populations. What we
can know of family planning around the world comes from a
number of sources: inferences from fertility statistics, which
in many instances are themselves faulty or incomplete; information about acceptance and practice from private and public programs set up to encourage family planning; the findings
of KAP surveys in which questions are asked about the
knowledge and use of contraceptives; records of manufacture
or sale of contraceptive materials and devices; hospital records
of admissions or diagnoses of abortion; health service records
from countries in which contraceptives or abortion services
are provided. There are some plausible estimates for some
countries made from sources such as these. But for many
countries there is no direct information.

Even though the extent of family planning remains unde-
termined, there seems to be agreement that it has been and
can be sufficiently extensive to affect the fertility of national
populations. Himes (1, p. 3, 4) has pointed out that ". . . widespread limitation of population by primitive peoples was an
established fact of ethnography and anthropology long before
Carr-Saunders [3] published his well-known and excellent
study." Noonan, on the basis of fragmentary evidence and
with allowance for other causes, decided that "it is not un-
reasonable to conclude that the fall in population [in Rome
in the third and fourth centuries] was also due to . . . the
deliberate avoidance of conception and childbearing" (2).
Although both present evidence of the existence of contraception in the Middle Ages, Noonan and Himes disagree
about its influence. Himes concluded, on the evidence available to him, that contraception was probably not sufficiently
used during the Middle Ages to have much of an effect on
population size. "The soundest conclusion," he wrote, "seems
to be that prior to late modern times, say 1800 in western

civilizations, much later in eastern civilizations, the numbers of a people on a given territory have been determined by various factors affecting natality and mortality, independently of attempts artificially to control conception" (1, p. 168). Although in no sense a social problem in Noonan's judgment, ". . . the practice of contraception was a reality of medieval civilization," and ". . . the demographic figures of the fourteenth and fifteenth centuries suggest that population control . . . occurred."

The decline in fertility that took place in Europe during the nineteenth and early part of the twentieth centuries was certainly influenced by factors other than deliberate attempts by organized groups to control conception. But it also occurred during a time when organized attempts to promote contraception appeared and spread widely and during a period of considerable advance in contraceptive techniques. Himes, whose work was originally published in 1936, said that about 200 mechanical devices—based on a few basic principles and varying only in details—were being used in Western cultures and that virtually all of them either originated or were improved in the nineteenth century. Wider use of the condom was facilitated by the invention of the technique of vulcanizing rubber; a rubber cervical cap was developed in 1838; the diaphragm was invented around 1881; a spermicidal paste or jelly appeared about the same time. It would seem unlikely that the combined influence of the spread of ideas and information, especially to the working classes, and the wider availability of improved methods of contraception played no part in the decline of birth rates. It seems more probable, especially in view of the relatively large geographical area involved, that the decline in birth rates in Europe and North America came about because people were changing socially and culturally and because a part of the change involved more extensive and more effective family planning.[1]

---

[1] A point of view with which most demographers would probably agree has been stated by Norman Ryder: "It may be asserted with confidence that fertility regulation, or the use of effective means to gain reproductive ends, is predominantly responsible for differences of fertility in time, in space, and between classes of population distinguished by socioeconomic and other criteria" (4).

If we can accept as evidence of extensive and effective family planning the ability of a national population with reasonably normal age distributions and no unusual patterns of age at marriage or proportions of married adults to achieve and maintain a crude birth rate of 25 or below, it is apparent that a substantial proportion of the world's population is and has been successfully practicing family planning. The December, 1965 *World Population Data Sheet* of the Population Reference Bureau, using largely United Nations data, lists 106 nations with populations of two million or over.[2] Of these, 31 nations with an aggregate estimated population of 1,024.5 millions (31 per cent of the estimated world population of 3.3 billion at mid-1965) have reported crude birth rates of under 25. These include every country in Europe[3] (except Iceland and Albania, neither of which is listed as having two million people); Canada and the United States in North America; Argentina and Uruguay in South America; Japan; Australia and New Zealand in Oceania; and the U.S.S.R. No African nation is included. For the most part, these countries achieved their low birth rates over a fairly long period of time, before oral contraceptives or the intra-uterine devices were available and before government contraceptive services were available. The development and growth of organizations to promote and popularize contraception that took place, especially in Europe and the United States, during the period of fertility decline probably had a considerable influence in opening up family planning as a topic for discussion and in stimulating the spread of information about contraceptives and their use. But the major force responsible for the decline must have been the development through time—in response to changing social, cultural, and economic conditions—of a climate of opinion favorable to the wide acceptance of a small family norm. Information,

---

[2] Unless otherwise specified, all figures used in this paper will refer to these nations, which have an aggregate population of 3,254.5 million, 98 per cent of the 3,308 million world population for mid-1965 as listed on the *World Population Data Sheet.*

[3] Ireland is included, but it is something of a special case since high age at marriage and the high proportion remaining unmarried could account for much of the low fertility.

216

motivation, and means occurring together contributed to a multitude of individual decisions and actions that collectively brought about and is maintaining low fertility.

Of the 106 countries with over two million people each, 57 have crude birth rates of 35 or over.[4] If a birth rate of 35 and over (and most of these countries are known or estimated to have rates above 40) can be considered evidence that family planning is not widely or effectively practiced, about two-thirds (66 per cent of the world's population live in countries where family planning is not yet sufficiently used to have a substantial effect on national fertility.[5] These countries include 13 in Latin America, 26 in Africa (31 if the countries for which no estimates are available are included), and 18 in Asia (including mainland China, 25 in Asia if the seven Asian countries for which estimates are not available are also included).

There are only six countries with two million or more population that have crude birth rates between 25 and 35: Cuba, Puerto Rico, Israel, Taiwan, and Hong Kong. Singapore probably belongs in this group, although its population in mid-1965 was estimated at just below two million. Puerto Rico and Hong Kong are not sovereign nations, and Puerto Rico is a special case in that its population composition and its fertility have been affected by opportunities for migration to the United States. Estimates for Cuba cover a range that could place it just above or just below a birth rate of 35. The birth rate for Israel is so close to 25 that it probably should be included among those countries that are successfully controlling fertility. Chile, Taiwan, Hong Kong, and Singapore are experiencing declining birth rates and there is presumptive evidence in all four countries that organized family

---

[4] This count includes mainland China, for which reliable information is not available but which probably has a birth rate in the high 30's. It does not include 12 additional countries with an estimated aggregate population of 101.3 million for which the *World Population Data Sheet* gives no information about fertility but which probably all have crude birth rates over 35: Lebanon, Saudi Arabia, Syria, and Yemen in the Middle East; Laos, North Vietnam, and North Korea in Asia; Ethiopia, Malawi, Somalia, Sierra Leone, and South Africa in Africa.

[5] The percentage is 64 if the 12 countries for which no fertility estimates are available are excluded; it falls to 42 per cent if mainland China is also excluded.

planning programs may be highly important contributing factors.

On the evidence of birth rates alone, then, it can be inferred that family planning is extensively and effectively practiced in all of Europe, in North America, in two (possibly three, if Chile is included) countries of South America, in Japan, in the large countries of Oceania, and in the U.S.S.R. In all of Africa, in all of Asia except Japan, Taiwan, Hong Kong, Singapore, and possibly mainland China—in most of Latin America, family planning is not yet sufficiently established to have had a large effect on fertility. These gross generalizations, of course, obscure many differences among and within countries in interest and activity relating to family planning.

If we turn to organized programs to promote the idea of family planning, we can note that these began in Europe in the nineteenth century, spread quickly to North America, and reached Asia in the second decade of the present century. In the past 20 years there has been a rapid expansion of such programs and they are now to be found on all continents. A Dutch Malthusian League (5) was formed in 1872; and the Dutch opened what is said to have been the world's first contraceptive clinic in 1878. England had a Malthusian League as early as 1876, and a French League for Human Regeneration was established in 1896. There was enough activity and movement in the U.S. as early as 1873 to stimulate the backlash efforts of Anthony Comstock and his Society for the Suppression of Vice, resulting in the enactment of the Comstock law that classified contraception as obscene and illegal and barred information about it from the U.S. mails. A First International Neo-Malthusian Conference was organized in France in 1900; a second and third followed at five-year intervals in Belgium and Holland, respectively, and a fourth was held in Germany in 1911. The United States got a National Birth Control League in 1915 and its first birth control clinic a year later. A Neo-Malthusian League was formed in India in 1916, according to the International Planned Parenthood Federation (Colonel B. F. Raina [6] says it appeared after 1925); a book on the population problem of India appeared in that same year. The New Culture

Movement in China endorsed birth control in 1919. In 1922 family planning activity began in Japan, and a clinic was opened in Hawaii. India had a clinic at Poona in 1923; the Labor Government of President Calles is said to have opened one in Mexico in 1925. In 1929 the government of Mysore opened the world's first government controlled family planning clinic. In 1927 the first World Population Conference was held in Switzerland and the International Union for the Scientific Investigation of Population Problems was founded. By 1940 there were family planning movements developed to the point of operating clinics in 19 countries, including five in Asia but none in Central or South America and none in Africa.

A quick, and possibly incomplete, count of present activity indicates that there are organized private family planning programs in some 58 countries of two million or more population that together include about 60 per cent of total world population. Of these, 34 are affiliated with the International Planned Parenthood Federation.[6] The IPPF operates from headquarters in London and through six regional offices and in 1966 had an operating budget in excess of two million dollars. It is presently supplying financial help to four Latin American countries whose organizations have not yet become affiliated.

Private programs are organized on all continents. Considering only those countries larger than two million population, family planning organizations are active in 17 countries of Asia, 16 in the Americas, 12 in Europe, 11 in Africa, and two in the Pacific area. In some countries they are just getting started; in others their programs remain weak and relatively ineffective; in some they are playing a major part in large-scale effective efforts to reduce national fertility.

In Taiwan, for example, which has one of the most successful of all family planning programs and one which seems to be having an effect on the birth rate, the action and service component of the nationwide program is handled by the voluntary Maternal and Child Health Association. The Planned Parenthood Federation of Korea, where there is also a suc-

---

[6] The IPPF also has affiliates in eight other countries with populations less than two million.

cessful national program, has supplemented the efforts of the National Family Planning Program, particularly in building public support, in the education and training of family planning workers, in the preparation and distribution of informational materials, and in the operation of mobile units. In Malaysia until the national program was started this year the Federation of Family Planning Associations was carrying on training and service programs in all the states of Malaya. The Singapore Family Planning Association, over a period of 16 years, built up a network of educational and service activities that certainly has had some influence in the decline in fertility which began in Singapore around 1957 and that laid the groundwork for the government program which began this year.

In a number of Latin American countries, voluntary organizations, usually with participation and frequently leadership from interested physicians, are moving to meet some of the demand for family planning information and services which is generating in that area. The Chilean National Association for Family Protection set in motion a series of events that have progressed to the point of government participation in large-scale family planning programs. The Honduras Association is collaborating with the Ministry of Health and AID in a program of expanding family planning services through public health facilities. The fledgling association in Colombia, as a part of its service, is receiving referrals from clinics at National University and the Jesuit Javeriana University and is providing intra-uterine devices for a rapidly increasing number of women in Bogota and other cities of the country. The Association for Family Welfare of Guatemala operates in three cities and gives some service to patients in the hospital which the government Social Security program operates in the capital. Costa Rica and El Salvador have recently established associations that are already finding a larger demand for services than they can supply. Bemfam, in Brazil, is rapidly moving toward the status of a national organization, with affiliates now active in a dozen cities and with plans for professional orientation and training and the development of a network of more than 50 satellite centers.

In Kenya it looks as though the government is going to authorize and support the Kenya Family Planning Association in a continuation and expansion of its existing training, public information, and service programs in lieu of more direct government activity in the immediate future. Private voluntary activity has been under way in the U.A.R. for a number of years, and until recently most of the available service—concentrated heavily in the Nile delta region from Cairo to Alexandria—was provided by private associations which continue to operate and attract a growing clientele. Private associations carry on all of the effective work in Rhodesia and South Africa; there are expanding associations in Nigeria and Sierra Leone, and there are the beginnings of an organized program even in Ethiopia.

The family planning movement has undoubtedly had a great deal to do with the rapid spread of population interest and activity throughout the world. There have been seven international conferences since 1946—six of them sponsored by the International Planned Parenthood Federation—and an eighth is being planned for Santiago, Chile in April of 1967. In addition, IPPF has organized 13 regional conferences since 1955 and four regional seminars since 1962. The latest of the seminars, held at Tegucigalpa, Honduras last June, was singularly successful in attracting medical and public health people from all over Latin America and in opening channels of communication among developing programs in that region.

The private organizations serve a number of important functions over and above the contraceptive service that they provide. They open the topic for public discussion and so help to legitimate it and to make it respectable. They both test out and create public opinion. They start information flowing through formal and informal channels. They bring issues into the open. They help to reduce political timidity. They bring to many people an awareness, often for the first time, that it is possible to have a choice about how many children will be born and when. They teach the benefits and the means of child spacing. They mobilize resources and leadership. And where private resources are inadequate to cope with the problems of ill health, family welfare, or economic

221

development arising from excess fertility, they become both groundbreakers for and stimulators of needed government efforts.

Although government interest in population and government attempts to influence it date back at least as far as early Roman times, large-scale, organized government fertility regulation programs are something new. There were none before 1950. Most of those that now exist were organized in the 1960's. Scorekeeping in this field is a little difficult because of uncertainties about how to define the beginning of a program and also because of certain ambiguities in the way governments have chosen to operate. The socialist countries of Eastern Europe, for example, certainly have what, viewed operationally, could be considered government programs, since both contraceptive and abortion services are provided through government facilities and by government personnel. As K. H. Mehlan put it at the Geneva conference, "In the socialist countries of Eastern Europe, all children are wanted children. Responsible parenthood is a basic ingredient of socialist health programs and of socialist population policy. . . . The reproductive behavior of the family in a socialist society develops in complete harmony between the individual and society. Marxists fear neither overpopulation nor underpopulation" (6). Thus there is no population policy (except the policy of having no policy), but there are numerous and effective family planning programs. In Taiwan, what is essentially an effective national program is defined as not a government program even though the government made funds available from interest on counterpart AID loans, permits its workers to engage in public education, and assures that its officers will direct the program through the device of having them serve also as officers of the Maternal and Child Health Association. (The Orient was never more inscrutable than this!) Japan has apparently had a government policy and program since 1952, but the program has been obscured by the conspicuous success of legalized abortion in contributing to continuing fertility decline after the passage of the Eugenic Protection Law in 1948. Therefore the government program is seldom heard of. India announced and began to organize a program as early as 1955, but it is only within the past year that the program has begun to gather any real momentum. Chile has a government supported program, but it is largely directed by university people and active mainly in Santiago. The United States cannot be said to have a government policy or program, although a number of federal and many state agencies are active in family planning.

Including mainland China, there are probably 13 countries that can be said to have national government programs. These include Chile in the Americas; Morocco, Tunisia, and the U.A.R. in North Africa; and in Asia: Turkey, Ceylon, India, Pakistan, Malaysia, Singapore, China, Japan, and South Korea. This is a list that anyone familiar with developments in this field can easily quarrel with. Taiwan, the country heralded as having the most innovative and effective of all national programs and certainly the best reported one, is not on it. Nor is Colombia, whose Minister of Health announced in September an appropriation of some five million pesos to the Colombian Association of Medical Faculties for a program to train all public health physicians in the country for family planning service. Peru is absent from the list, although a presidential decree of a couple of years ago established a new Center for Population and Development Studies to be a joint activity of the Ministries of Labor and Health. Missing too is the United States, which is actively supporting family planning programs both here and abroad and which is actually operating one in the health department of the District of Columbia and several for special populations such as the military and Indian groups. Also missing are the socialist countries of Eastern Europe, including the U.S.S.R.

Of the countries on the list, Japan alone has low fertility. This is probably due less to the effects of the government program or policy than to the operating of "spontaneous" factors similar to those that were influencing fertility in Europe and the U.S. from the middle of the nineteenth century. In Japan these factors produced both a high level of motivation for small families and convenient means, through abortion and contraception, to make them possible, and the result was a birth rate that dropped rapidly from levels that were not very high at any time in the postwar years.

Taiwan, Chile, and Singapore have moderate fertility. In Taiwan the crude birth rate has been dropping since 1955. How much of the recent decline is due to the national program started in 1964 and the extensive activity of prepregnancy health workers dating from 1959 can only be estimated, but it is highly probable that the decline reflects more and possibly better family planning by couples in the population. The Chilean rate seems to have remained fairly constant from 1930 to 1960 and has apparently dropped slightly since. What, if any, part of the decline is attributable to the family planning program is a matter for speculation. Singapore has had a declining birth rate since 1957. The Singapore Family Planning Association has claimed some credit for the decline, but a professor of demography at Singapore University has argued that the fall was almost entirely due to other causes.

All of the other countries on the list (with China being uncertain but probably to be included) have high fertility, as defined by a crude birth rate of 35 or higher. India's program is the oldest of this group, but the problem of India is massive, there were few or no guidelines for the country to follow, much of the history of the country's program took place before oral contraceptives and the IUD were widely available, and the program suffered from the beginning from not having a high enough status in the government. There is some evidence that many of the administrative problems are being overcome and that the program is now beginning to move. Certainly the more recent reports coming out of the country are more heartening than earlier ones. The problem remains both incredibly complex and massive, but there are grounds for new hope that it can be handled. Pakistan started its program in 1960 and reorganized it almost entirely in 1964 to 1965. The administrative structure was strengthened and tightened; training, research, and service components were expanded; new, modest numerical targets were established. The new program has not been in operation long enough to have had much of an effect. The Korean program, started in 1964 with principal reliance on IUD's, has expanded rapidly and by the end of 1965 reported about 350,000 insertions. Numerical targets are being met; careful records are kept; evaluation procedures are well developed. This gives promise of being an effective program. The programs of Tunisia, Turkey, Ceylon, Malaysia, Morocco, and the U.A.R. are too recent or still too undeveloped for much to be said about their prospects. At this stage what is most important is not the effect on fertility, but that there are 13 governments that, largely in the past ten years, have adopted population policies and are backing them up with family planning programs.

In addition to the 13 countries that have national policies and programs, there are some 30 others in which the governments or some of their departments or branches are active or involved in family planning. The degree of activity or involvement ranges all the way from the large and varied activities of the U.S. government, domestic and international, to permitting a private organization to work in a single government facility, as is occurring in Guatemala. In Honduras, for example, there is active collaboration between the Ministry of Health and the voluntary family planning organization in the operation of a program of service and information. In Mexico, hospitals of the Social Security program are experimenting with IUD insertions in a program designed to learn whether and how induced abortions can be reduced. The Peruvian Center for Population and Development Studies last year sponsored a conference on population problems, addressed at one time or another by the President of the Republic and the Minister of Health, at which the need for family planning programs was openly advocated. Venezuela has a population office in the Ministry of Health that has proposed trial programs in Caracas and other cities. In Kenya government facilities are used by the Family Planning Association for both training and service activities. A Population Council mission, invited by the government of Kenya, has prepared a set of recommendations on family planning which have been favorably received by the government. Algeria is undertaking a national knowledge-attitude-practice survey to find out what its people think, know, and do about fertility. In Nigeria, the university and the health department at Lagos are collaborating in a family planning program. Iran has requested that a mission from the Population Council study its problem and advise it about a possible family planning program. The municipal health department in Manila is quietly offering family planning service in sections of that city. Thailand has conducted a rural experiment in family planning, with help from the Population Council and the University of Michigan, and contraceptive service is now being offered in one or more municipal clinics in Bangkok. In Norway, Switzerland, and the United Kingdom, some family planning services are offered in government clinics, and in the European socialist countries, as noted earlier, governments generally provide a wide range of contraceptive and abortion services.[7]

In some 26 countries governments directly support family planning or related organizations either through direct subsidies or under contractual arrangements for services such as training. These include three countries in the Americas (the U.S., Chile, and Colombia), five in Africa (Nigeria, South Africa, Kenya, Rhodesia, U.A.R.), ten in Asia (Turkey, Ceylon, Nepal, Pakistan, Malaysia, Thailand, Taiwan, Hong Kong, South Korea, Singapore), seven in Europe (Denmark, Finland, West Germany, Sweden, United Kingdom, East Germany, Poland), and one (New Zealand) in the Pacific.

In world perspective, legal or liberal abortion policies are important aspects of family planning. No country in the Americas, Africa, or the Pacific region has such policies. Two countries in Asia—Japan and, probably, mainland China—do. Twelve European countries have them, including all the socialist countries of Eastern Europe, Yugoslavia, the U.S.S.R., and Denmark, Finland, Sweden, and Switzerland in Northern and Western Europe. Something of the effect of abortion in family planning can be seen in figures presented by Dr. Christopher Tietze (7) at the American Public Health Association meeting in San Francisco in November, 1966. In the last year (1962) for which data were presented for the three northern countries, Sweden, Denmark, and Finland, the ratio of abortions to each 1,000 live births was respectively 30, 51, and 74. The latest figures available for six

---

[7] This is an area of such rapid change that any of these comments may be outdated before they are printed.

socialist countries for years ranging from 1959 to 1965 varied from a low of 250 legal abortions for each 1,000 live births in Yugoslavia (1961) through 630 in Bulgaria (1963) to 1,400 in Hungary (1964). In Japan, where the number of abortions was rapidly increasing even before the liberal Eugenic Protection Law in 1948, reported abortions rose to 1.17 millions in 1955. The trend has been downward since then but not as rapidly as had been hoped. Factors in the continuing popularity of abortion—in Japan as well as elsewhere where it is legal—are its low cost, the case with which it can be obtained, its safety when done under medical auspices, its effectiveness in preventing unwanted births, and its usefulness in correcting contraceptive failures.

Excluding mainland China, countries with liberal abortion policies include some 470 million people, about 14 per cent of world population. If China is included, the population totals around 1,180 million—about 36 per cent of the world total.

Even in many countries where abortion laws are restrictive or prohibitive, it is likely that abortion is a widely used form of family planning. Survey and other research data from such countries as Chile, Colombia, Peru, South Korea, and Taiwan indicate a considerable incidence of induced abortion. The data are generally of two kinds: responses of women to questions about their own pregnancy experiences and studies of admissions to hospitals for incomplete or septic abortions. Both the results and the methods of reporting them vary from study to study, but almost all show that abortion is common. Reasonably typical are the results of several surveys in Chile (6, 8) which show that about a quarter of the women questioned indicated that they had deliberately terminated one or more pregnancies. Hospital studies in that country indicated that in the period 1958–1960, abortions accounted for 27 per cent of admissions to National Health Service hospitals and 29 per cent of all bed-days in those hospitals. Korean reports show about the same proportion of abortions; those from Taiwan indicate somewhat less. In Chile and Mexico experimental studies are being undertaken to see whether the number of induced abortions can be reduced by providing effective contraceptive methods to women at risk.

In Latin America, in particular, there is a growing interest in the problems of abortion and it is likely that additional studies and experiments to reduce the number of dangerous and costly illegal abortions will be undertaken.

Abortion, as Ronald Freedman said in his summary of the Geneva conference, "may be the most widely used single method (of family limitation) in the world today" (6). Legal or illegal, it is a huge worldwide phenomenon that needs much more attention than it has received.

Perhaps the most meaningful way to sum up the family planning picture is by geographic region. (The following considers only those countries shown on the *World Population Data Sheet* as having populations of two million or more at mid-1965).

Americas

Northern America: Both countries of North America, with a total population of 214.2 million, are effectively practicing family planning. Neither can be said to have a national government program, although the United States has perhaps come close to having one in the past two years. Canada has some legal restrictions on family planning; on the other hand there are services offered in some local government facilities. Both countries have active private programs affiliated with IPPF.

Middle America: Cuba and Puerto Rico are exceptions to the pattern in this region. Each has a crude birth rate between 25 and 35. Puerto Rico is an exceptional case because of extensive migration to the U.S., which may have affected the age structure of the population. There have also been extensive efforts to introduce contraception there. Cuba may have enough family planning to be starting through the fertility transition, but information from the island is meager. All other countries in the region have high fertility. There are no national government programs. In five countries, El Salvador, Guatemala, Honduras, Mexico, Puerto Rico, family planning services are being offered in one or more government facilities with either a service or research justification. Six countries have active family associations. Those of Mexico and Puerto Rico are affiliated with IPPF. Those of El Salvador, Guatemala, and Costa Rica (which has fewer than two million population) receive financial help from both IPPF and AID. There is likely to be a rapid increase of interest and activity in El Salvador, Honduras, and Costa Rica, and possibly in Mexico.

South America: Two countries, Argentina and Uruguay, are effectively limiting fertility. None of the others is, although the Chilean birth rate is in the 25 to 35 range and may now be coming down, partly as a result of increased family planning activity. Chile can be considered to have a national government program, although much of the initiative remains in the hands of university faculty people and there is not much activity outside of Santiago. The Minister of Health of Colombia in September was quoted in Colombian newspapers as saying the country will have a national program which will begin with a training program under which the Colombian Association of Faculties of Medicine will train all public health physicians for family planning. All universities in Colombia have interdisciplinary committees concerned with family planning; all are conducting some type of family planning or demographic research, some of which includes service clinics. Peru and Venezuela have government agencies devoted to population matters. In Chile and Colombia government funds have gone into support of programs of either service or training conducted by private or quasi-governmental organizations. All countries in the region except Bolivia and Venezuela have family planning associations. (Bolivia may have by now.) That of Chile is affiliated with IPPF. Those in Colombia and Brazil are receiving funds from IPPF. Expansion of interest and activity in the near future is most likely to occur in Brazil and Colombia. There are legal restrictions on the distribution of contraceptive materials or information in Brazil, Colombia, Ecuador, Paraguay, and Uruguay.

Europe

Northern and Western Europe: Every country in the area is successfully limiting its fertility. There are no national government programs, although in Denmark, Finland, West Germany, United Kingdom, and Sweden the government contributes to the support of private family planning associations, and government facilities are used for family planning information and service in Norway, Switzerland, and the United Kingdom. There are legal restrictions in Austria (the same type as apply to other drugs), Belgium, France, West Germany, Iceland, and the Netherlands. A movement to try to get the French laws changed failed in 1956; according to newspaper reports in November, 1966, another attempt was being made.[8] Abortion is legal or liberal in Denmark, Finland, Sweden, and Switzerland. A West German law was repealed in 1960. There is considerable sterilization reported in Switzerland. All countries except Austria, Iceland, and Norway have family planning associations. The Switzerland association operates only in one canton, Vaud. All of the associations except the one in West Germany are affiliated with IPPF.

Eastern Europe: Every country in the region has low fertility, indicating effective family planning. There are no national programs, although the government provides abortion and contraception services or supports private associations in all countries. Government departments offer family planning service in Czechoslovakia, East Germany, and Romania; government support to private associations is given in Poland and East Germany, the only two countries that have them. The Polish association is affiliated with IPPF. Abortion is liberal or legal in all countries.

Southern Europe: All countries effectively limit fertility. There are no national government programs, although services are given in government facilities in Yugoslavia, where abortion is legal. There are legal restrictions on family planning in Italy, Portugal, and Spain. Italy has a private family planning association.

U.S.S.R.: Fertility is low, indicating successful family planning. There is no official announced program, but contraception and abortion services are readily available through government facilities. Abortion is legal.

---

[8] It failed.

Oceania: Both Australia and New Zealand have low fertility. Each has a private association affiliated with IPPF. There are no national government programs, but New Zealand provides financial support for the private association.

Africa

Northern and Eastern Africa: No country has effective family planning. There are national government programs in Morocco (just starting), Tunisia, and the U.A.R. Government departments or agencies are active in population or family planning to some extent in Algeria, Kenya, Rhodesia, Uganda, and the U.A.R. Some financial support is provided by the government to private associations in Kenya, Rhodesia, and the U.A.R. There are private associations in eight countries; three are affiliated with IPPF. Zambia has had a private association, but does not have one now. It receives some services from the association in Rhodesia. There are probably legal restrictions in four countries; a restrictive law in Tunisia was repealed in 1961.

Western, Middle, and Southern Africa: There is no family planning effective enough to bring birth rates down. This is an area of relatively little interest or activity. There are no national government programs. Nigeria has a program operating in part through the health department in Lagos. There are private associations in Nigeria, Sierra Leone, and South Africa. South Africa is affiliated with IPPF. Nigeria and South Africa provide some government support to private activity. All countries except Ghana, Nigeria, Sierra Leone, and South Africa probably have restrictive legislation.

Asia

Southwest Asia: There is little demographic information available on fertility in this area. What there is indicates that probably no country—with the possible exception of Israel—is successfully limiting fertility. Israel has moderate to low fertility with a crude birth rate just above 25. Turkey has the only national government program in the region. Jordan permits some activity in a government facility. Israel, Jor-

231

dan, and Turkey have private associations; Jordan and Turkey provide some government support to theirs, which are affiliated with IPPF.

Middle South Asia: Fertility remains high in all countries despite considerable government and private family planning activity. There are national government programs in Ceylon, India, and Pakistan. Iran has asked for a survey mission from the Population Council and is said to be offering some services through facilities of the Ministry of Health. There are associations in all countries except Afghanistan; those of Ceylon, India, Nepal, and Pakistan are affiliated with IPPF. Ceylon, Nepal, and Pakistan provide some government support to the private associations. India has probably the largest and most active national program in the world. It had what is said to have been the first government clinic in the world in Mysore in 1930; in July, 1965, it was reported to have some 15,800 family planning units operating as well as 3,200 sterilization units. Its target for IUD's for the current year is four million insertions.[9]

South East Asia: All countries have high fertility. There is one national government program, in Malaysia. (Singapore also has one but was not listed as having two million people at mid-1965). Services are offered in some government facilities in Indonesia, the Philippines, and Thailand. There are private associations in Burma, Indonesia, Malaysia, the Philippines, and Thailand. All except Indonesia are affiliated with IPPF. There are legal restrictions in Burma.

East Asia: Japan is the only low fertility country in the area. Birth rates in Taiwan and Hong Kong are in the middle range and appear to be falling. These (together with Singapore) may be the first successes to be reported for deliberate attempts to reduce fertility in developing countries. Japan and South Korea have national government programs; China probably does also. Taiwan has a successful national program, but it is not carried on as an official government activity. Government personnel and facilities are used by the program in Taiwan. Japan and China (probably) have legal abortion. There are private associations in Taiwan,

[9] The accomplishment was just over one million insertions in 1966.

Hong Kong, Japan, and South Korea. All except that in Taiwan are affiliated with IPPF. Government funds help support private activities in Taiwan, Hong Kong, and South Korea.

Looking at the world picture from the viewpoint of the urgent need to bring population growth under control, there are grounds for both pessimism and optimism. Two-thirds of the world's population are not yet effectively limiting their fertility, and for a good proportion of them there are not yet many indications that they soon will. There are nine high fertility countries, with over 20 million population each, that do not yet have either national programs or reasonably effective private ones on a large scale. These are Iran, Burma, Indonesia, Thailand, and the Philippines in Asia; Ethiopia and Nigeria in Africa; Mexico and Brazil in Latin America. Iran is moving toward what may become a national program. Burma remains largely cut off from the rest of the world and is probably not likely soon to take any action. Indonesia, the largest of them all with over 105 million people, may move rapidly toward the creation of programs as it stabilizes politically. Recent news from the Philippines indicates a strong tendency to put its reliance on improving agricultural productivity. There is activity in Thailand, where a most successful rural demonstration was held and where there have been long lines of people in Bangkok waiting for service; but the government does not have a national program. There is not a great deal of official sentiment favorable to family planning in Ethiopia. The prospects would be better in Nigeria if there were a more stable governmental structure. There is emerging concern in both Brazil and Mexico, and either may move rapidly toward large-scale program efforts.

It has not yet been clearly demonstrated that population growth can be achieved by deliberate programs in advance of the changes in social and economic conditions associated with low fertility in the developed countries. There are promising indications, but the definitive answer is not yet in.

On the other hand, interest in population and programs to help alleviate its pressures are growing even faster than population. Fertility surveys show a wide receptivity to the idea of family planning and a widely expressed preference for fewer children. Over a dozen governments have instituted national programs in the past ten years, most of them in the past five, and more than a dozen others have taken positive actions of one type or another. Two governments—the United States and Sweden—are heavily committed in their foreign aid programs to support of efforts to reduce population growth; Sweden gives it top priority. A third government—Great Britain—provides some limited support for overseas population programs in the Commonwealth area. The United Nations Population Division is moving steadily closer to an active interest in family planning; two of the UN member organizations, WHO and UNICEF, have considered a more active role in family planning programs; FAO has warned of the growing imbalance between population and food supply and has strongly urged more effective family planning; the Economic Commission for Asia and the Far East (ECAFE) has sponsored a regional seminar on family planning administration and is considering one on information programs for family planning. The Pan American Union will sponsor a population conference in Caracas next spring. Professional schools of medicine and, to a lesser extent, nursing and social work are preparing students for participation in family planning; schools of public health have developed programs to train personnel for family planning program administration and operation and are active in relevant research both in the United States and abroad. Private foundations, such as Ford and Rockefeller, are active in support of research, training, and action demonstration programs in many countries. The Ford Foundation, for example, presently has 33 persons doing full-time professional work in population, 26 of whom are working in developing countries; to date the Foundation has made population grants totaling more than $73 million. The Population Council is active in biological and demographic research and training and provides technical assistance to a number of government programs. There is a growing cadre of professional people with a full-time commitment to family planning.

About a third of the world's population is already successfully limiting its fertility and did so before the oral and intra-uterine contraceptives were available, indicating how powerful the desire for smaller families can be when it spreads to a country or region. The acceptability and effectiveness of the new contraceptives have been such as to give a powerful stimulus to both private and public programs. There are promising new contraceptive methods in the offing that will be cheaper, easier to use, and even more effective than those now known. Over much of the world, reproduction and family planning can now be talked about more openly and in more circumstances than ever before.

Family planning as a social movement has developed enormous vitality, large human and technical resources, and strong momentum. It has grown partly in response to an increasing awareness of the urgent challenge with which mankind is confronted, partly out of a humanistic concern for the health, welfare, and dignity of women, children, and families. In one form or another family planning has been around for a long time. It will not diminish. It will persist; it will grow. If we are fortunate, it may reach a level of acceptance and effectiveness high enough to make a difference in the quality of life a few generations from now.

REFERENCES

1. Himes, Norman E. *Medical History of Contraception.* New York: Gamut Press, 1963.
2. Noonan, John T., Jr. *Contraception: A History of Its Treatment by the Catholic Theologians and Canonists.* Cambridge: Harvard University Press, 1965.
3. Carr-Saunders, A. M. *The Population Problem.* Oxford: Clarendon Press, 1922.
4. Ryder, N. B. "Fertility." In Philip Hauser and Otis Dudley Duncan, eds., *The Study of Population: An Inventory and Appraisal.* Chicago: University of Chicago Press, 1959.
5. International Planned Parenthood Federation. *Historical Highlights of Birth Control: Malthus (1798) to Tokyo, Japan (1955).* IPPF, undated.
6. Berelson, Bernard, *et al.,* eds. *Family Planning and Population Programs.* Chicago: University of Chicago Press, 1966.
7. Tietze, Christopher. "Abortions in Europe." Unpublished

paper presented at the American Public Health Association meeting, San Francisco, October 31–November 4, 1966.

8. Armijo, Rolando and Requena, Mariano. "Epidemiological Aspects of Abortion." Unpublished paper presented at the American Public Health Association meeting, San Francisco, October 31–November 4, 1966.

TABLE 1 Family Planning Status Summary, 106 Countries with Populations of Two Million or Over, by Geographic Region

Region	Number of Countries	Aggregate Population (millions)	Per Cent of Aggregate Total Population
Have effective family planning as indicated by a C.B.R. of 25 or less:			
North America	2	214.2	
Latin America	2	25.1	
Africa	0	—	
Asia	1	97.8	
Europe	23	439.3	
U.S.S.R.	1	234.0	
Oceania	2	14.1	
Totals	31	1,024.5	31%
Have ineffective family planning as indicated by a C.B.R. of 35 or more:			
North America	0	—	
Latin America	13	187.0	
Africa	26*	242.2*	
Asia (other than China)	17*	951.8*	
China	1	710.0	
Europe	0	—	
Oceania	0	—	
Totals	57	2,091.0	64%
Have moderately effective family planning as indicated by C.B.R.'s between 25 and 35† or no information is available:			
Latin America	3	18.9	
Africa	5	49.1	
Asia	10	71.0	
Totals	18	139.0	4%
Countries that have national government programs:‡			
Latin America (Chile)	1	8.7	
Africa (Morocco, Tunisia, U. A. R.)	3	47.6	
Asia (Turkey, Ceylon, India, Pakistan, Malaysia, China, Japan, Korea)	8	1,485.9	
Totals	12	1,542.2	47%

* There are five countries in Africa (Ethiopia, Malawi, Somalia, Sierra Leone, and South Africa) with an aggregate population of 49.1 million and seven in Asia (Lebanon, Saudi Arabia, Syria, Yemen, Laos, North Vietnam, and North Korea) with an aggregate population of 52.2 million for which C.B.R. information is not available. It is likely that all have high fertility. If all were added to the above breakdown, there would be 69 countries with an aggregate population of 2140.1 million constituting 66 per cent of the total.

† There are only six countries in this category: Cuba, Puerto Rico, Chile, Israel, Taiwan, and Hong Kong.

‡ Taiwan perhaps should be included here since its program seems to be a government one in everything but name. Singapore also has a national government program but its population in mid-1965 was estimated at slightly under two million.

Family Planning and Economic Development

TABLE 1 Family Planning Status Summary, 106 Countries with Populations of Two Million or Over, by Geographic Region (Cont'd)

Region	Number of Countries	Aggregate Population (millions)	Per Cent of Aggregate Total Population
Countries that have organized private family planning programs:			
North America	2	214.2	
Latin America	14	207.2	
Africa	11	181.3	
Asia	17	1,022.4	
Europe	12	305.0	
Oceania	2	14.1	
Totals	58	1944.2	60%

TABLE 2 Family Planning Status Summary, 106 Countries with Populations of Two Million or Over

	Estimated population, mid-1965 (millions)	C.B.R. 25 or less	C.B.R 35 or more	C.B.R. between 25 and 35 (M) or not available (NA)	National government program	One or more government agencies or departments engaged in family planning or population activity or research	Government financial support to private organizations	Abortion legal or liberal abortion laws	Organized private program	IPPF affiliate (x) or receives IPPF funds (F)
AMERICA										
Northern America										
Canada	19.6	x				x			x	x
U.S.	194.6	x				x	x		x	x
Middle America										
Cuba	7.6			M						
Dominican Republic	3.6		x						x	
El Salvador	2.9		x			x			x	F
Guatemala	4.4		x			x			x	F
Haiti	4.7		x						x	
Honduras	2.2		x			x			x	x
Mexico	40.9		x			x			x	
Puerto Rico	2.6			M		x			x	x
South America										
Argentina	22.4	x							x	
Bolivia	3.7		x						x	
Brazil	81.3		x						x	F
Chile	8.7			M	x		x		x	x
Colombia	15.8		x			x	x		x	F
Ecuador	5.1		x						x	
Paraguay	2.0		x						x	
Peru	11.7		x				x		x	
Uruguay	2.7	x							x	
Venezuela	8.7		x			x				

Sources: Grouping of countries, population, birth rates are from the Population Reference Bureau, *World Population Data Sheet,* December, 1965. Other information is from a variety of sources including particularly the report of the 1965 Geneva Conference, *Family Planning and Population Programs,* and a January, 1966 report of IPPF, "Family Planning in Five Continents." The time of reference is mid-1965 for demographic data and the years 1965 and 1966 for other information. The data are as complete and accurate as they could be made in the time available. There may be omissions, and with fast changing conditions any item could soon be outdated.

TABLE 2   Family Planning Status Summary, 106 Countries with Populations of Two Million or Over—(Cont'd)

	Estimated population, mid-1965 (millions)	C.B.R. 25 or less	C.B.R 35 or more	C.B.R. between 25 and 35 (M) or not available (NA)	National government program	One or more government agencies or departments engaged in family planning or population activity or research	Government financial support to private organizations	Abortion legal or liberal abortion laws	Organized private program	IPPF affiliate (x) or receives IPPF funds (F)
EUROPE										
Northern and Western Europe										
Austria	7.3	x								
Belgium	9.4	x							x	x
Denmark	4.8	x					x	x	x	x
Finland	4.6	x					x	x	x	x
France	48.8	x							x	x
W. Germany	56.8	x					x		x	x
Ireland	2.8	x								
Netherlands	12.3	x							x	x
Norway	3.7	x				x				
Sweden	7.7	x					x	x	x	x
Switzerland	6.0	x					x	x	x	x
United Kingdom	54.4	x					x	x	x	x
Eastern Europe										
Bulgaria	8.2	x						x		
Czechoslovakia	14.2	x				x		x		
E. Germany	16.0	x				x	x	x	x	
Hungary	10.1	x						x		
Poland	31.6	x					x	x	x	x
Romania	19.1	x				x		x		
Southern Europe										
Greece	8.6	x								
Italy	52.6	x							x	
Portugal	9.2	x								
Spain	31.6	x								
Yugoslavia	19.5	x				x		x		
OCEANIA										
Australia	11.4	x							x	x
New Zealand	2.7	x					x		x	x
U.S.S.R.	234.0	x				x		x		

TABLE 2 Family Planning Status Summary, 106 Countries with Populations of Two Million or Over—(Cont'd)

	Estimated population, mid-1965 (millions)	C.B.R. 25 or less	C.B.R. 35 or more	C.B.R. between 25 and 35 (M) or not available (NA)	National government program	One or more government agencies or departments engaged in family planning or population activity or research	Government financial support to private organizations	Abortion legal or liberal abortion laws	Organized private program	IPPF affiliate (x) or receives IPPF funds (F)
AFRICA										
Northern and Eastern Africa										
Algeria	12.6	x				x				
Burundi	2.9	x								
Ethiopia	22.6			NA					x	
Kenya	9.4	x				x	x		x	x
Madagascar	6.4	x							x	
Malawi	4.0			NA						
Morocco	13.3	x			x					
Rhodesia	4.3	x				x	x		x	
Rwanda	3.1	x								
Somalia	2.4			NA						
Sudan	13.5	x							x	
Tanzania	10.6	x							x	
Tunisia	4.7	x			x					
Uganda	7.6	x				x			x	x
U.A.R. (Egypt)	29.6	x			x	x	x		x	x
Zambia	3.7	x							?	
Western, Middle, and Southern Africa										
Angola	5.2	x								
Cameroon	5.2	x								
Chad	3.4	x								
Congo (Leopoldville)	15.6	x								
Dahomey	2.4	x								
Ghana	7.9	x								
Guinea	3.5	x								
Ivory Coast	3.8	x								
Mali	4.6	x								
Niger	3.4	x								
Nigeria	57.2	x				x	x		x	
Senegal	3.5	x								
Sierra Leone	2.2			NA					x	
South Africa	17.9			NA			x		x	x
Upper Volta	4.8	x								

241

TABLE 2   Family Planning Status Summary, 106 Countries with Populations of Two Million or Over—(Cont'd)

	Estimated population, mid-1965 (millions)	C.B.R. 25 or less	C.B.R. 35 or more	C.B.R. between 25 and 35 (M) or not available (NA)	National government program	One or more government agencies or departments engaged in family planning or population activity or research	Government financial support to private organizations	Abortion legal or liberal abortion laws	Organized private program	IPPF affiliate (x) or receives IPPF funds (F)
ASIA										
South West Asia										
Iraq	7.8		x							
Israel	2.6			M					x	
Jordan	2.0		x			x			x	x
Lebanon	2.3			NA						
Saudi Arabia	6.8			NA						
Syria	5.6			NA						
Turkey	31.6		x		x		x		x	x
Yemen	5.0			NA						
Middle South Asia										
Afghanistan	15.6		x							
Ceylon	11.2		x		x		x		x	x
India	482.5		x		x				x	x
Iran	23.4		x			x			x	
Nepal	10.1		x				x		x	x
Pakistan	115.0		x		x		x		x	x
South East Asia										
Burma	24.7		x						x	x
Cambodia	6.4		x							
Indonesia	104.6		x			x			x	
Laos	2.0			NA						
Malaysia	9.4		x		x		x		x	x
Philippines	32.3		x			x			x	x
Thailand	30.6		x			x	x		x	x
N. Vietnam	18.5			NA						
S. Vietnam	16.2		x							
East Asia										
China (Mainland)	710.0			NA	x				x	
China (Taiwan)	12.4			M	x	x			x	
Hong Kong	3.8			M			x		x	x
Japan	97.8	x			x			x	x	x
N. Korea	12.0			NA						
S. Korea	28.4		x		x		x		x	x

TABLE 3   Estimated Crude Birth Rates, Gross Reproduction Rates, and Completed Family Size for the Regions of the World

(Weighted averages of most recently available rates for countries within each region)

Region	Crude Birth Rate	Gross Repro-duction Rate	Completed Family Size[1]
World Total[2]	34–36	2.2–2.3	4.5–4.7
Developing Regions[2]	40–43	2.6–2.7	5.3–5.5
Africa	48	3.0	6.1
North Africa	46	2.9	5.9
West Africa	54	3.4	7.0
South & East Africa	45	2.7	5.5
Asia (excluding U.S.S.R.)[2]	39–42	2.5–2.7	5.1–5.5
South West Asia	45	3.0	6.1
South Central Asia	44	2.9	5.9
South East Asia	49	2.9	5.9
East Asia[2]	32–39	2.1–2.5	4.3–5.1
Middle & South America	41	2.8	5.7
Middle America	45	3.0	6.1
South America	40	2.7	5.5
More Developed Regions	22	1.4	2.9
Northern America	24	1.8	3.7
Europe	19	1.3	2.7
Northern & Western Europe	18	1.3	2.7
Central Europe	18	1.2	2.5
Southern Europe	20	1.2	2.5
Oceania	24	1.8	3.7
U.S.S.R.	25	1.4	2.9

[1] Average number of children born per woman living through the reproductive period.
[2] Range of estimated values corresponding to alternative estimates for mainland China.
Source: W. Parker Mauldin, "Fertility Studies: Knowledge, Attitude, and Practice." *Studies in Family Planning*, no. 7, June, 1965.

DISCUSSION

A need for further research in the area of population has been stressed by both Ronald Freedman and Julian Samora in their discussions of Lyle Saunders' paper, "Family Planning, the Worldwide View." A strong feeling that research is a prerequisite to efficient alleviation of population problems was expressed. Mr. Samora cautions persons who are optimistic about the present progress of such programs. He questions Mr. Saunders about the practicality and effectiveness of the present family planning programs scattered throughout the world. Mr. Freedman emphasizes the complexity of the human and the multimotivational forces behind every human action. He suggests that these motivations be studied to avoid attribution of an action to a false cause.

FREEDMAN: I think Lyle Saunders has given a well-balanced view of the situation. He has tried to stress both optimism and pessimism. But the kind of paper he gives necessarily stresses optimism, because it calls to attention all the things that are being done organizationally. However, the question is: How effective are these programs in helping the masses of the population interested in birth control? In view of a necessarily optimistic bias in the kind of presentation Mr. Saunders gave, I am going to give my pessimistic view. Based on close observation of half a dozen or so of these major programs, I would like to stress that once a program is begun it becomes very complex and difficult, and there are going to be some bad days. I think this year in many ways is a bad year. A lot of problems have arisen now which have to be faced realistically, otherwise persons will become demoralized, depressed, and give up. This has happened in a number of cases. My long-run view is basically optimistic, but I would like to stress some of the problems.

Mr. Saunders was right, I believe, in describing the program in Taiwan as very good. I am associated with it, but I can not take any credit for it. It is being run by a group of very good Chinese doctors and social scientists who are doing an excellent job. But let me mention illustratively some aspects of the situation. The birth rate has been declining, as Mr. Saunders pointed out. We still do not know whether the program, though successful by some criteria, has made much difference. Perhaps the birth rate would have declined even without the program. We do not know to what extent the program is substituting program services for that which would have been done anyway. We do know, for example, that a lot of the persons accepting the program services were using contraception or abortion outside of the program. Now, from a welfare, humanistic point of view, I believe this leaves much to be desired, irrespective of its effect on the birth rate. It is better to convince persons to give up abortion for a more suitable method or a more secure contraceptive method. But we do not know the extent to which this is being done.

So far as I know, in every one of the countries with a major intra-uterine device program which has had a big start, there has been a decline in the number of insertions. In last year's Taiwan program there were more than 99,500 insertions. The goal was 100,000. This year the goal was 120,000; I think they will make 90,000. They were getting about 10,000 to 12,000 a month. This number has been reduced to 7,000, though surveys indicate that 50 per cent or more of the women in the childbearing years do not want more children. The reason for this decline is very complex.

Korea: Korea has an excellent program. They have inserted about 400,000 intra-uterine devices. It increased to 40-some thousand a month about six months ago. It is now down to about 20,000, although all expectations were that it would take off from that point. In every one of the countries in which we have had experience, a substantial number of women who have had the IUD inserted no longer have it in place after about 18 months.

245

We have very good data on this for Taiwan. They inserted many IUD's, but 60 per cent of them are now out, according to a report which I saw last week.

Hong Kong: The birth rate has been falling rapidly in Hong Kong. Half of that decline is due to a distortion in the age structure and has nothing to do with birth control. The IUD program has fallen off there, just as it has in other places. The number of insertions is down, and the removal rate is up.

Singapore: As Mr. Saunders indicated, there is real doubt as to what is at work there.

India: I do not think anybody, including the Indians, knows what is going on in India, and that is one of the depressing facts. Many persons are inserting IUD's, but they do not know exactly how many have been inserted, nor do they know how many have been taken out, although in a report I received about a month ago the rate of removal in the 12 New Delhi clinics had begun to exceed the rate of insertion. That is not good, and since they have not been doing a follow-up, they do not know why this is happening.

I can not help mentioning the United States, since Mr. Saunders took the countries with birth rates below 25 and said they had effective family planning. I want to remind you that about 20 per cent of the women ages 35 to 39 interviewed in the United States said that they had more children than they wanted. In a longitudinal study in Detroit, we have talked to women who had a fourth baby four years ago. Sixty per cent of them said either that baby or the one after it was an unwanted child. This a rather pessimistic set of circumstances. I think something can be done about it along the lines of Mr. Saunders' comments at the end of his paper. I have ideas and I am sure you have ideas of what is involved. This is a complicated matter and is not solved simply by making contraceptives available. It is a very complex motivational problem.

In most of the underdeveloped countries the people really mean what they say in the surveys. Usually about 50 or 60 per cent of women in the childbearing years say they do not want more children. But that is only one motivation and humans, being complex, have many. They are in a state of ambivalence. They want more effective family planning today, maybe they do not tomorrow. They want this, but they are worried about whether their children will really live because they are from a tradition of high mortality. They are also worried about the opinions of others.

A massive support and legitimation of this activity is required. One rather interesting research finding from our work in Taiwan supports this idea. We find that Taiwanese people who believe that their friends, relatives, and neighbors are practicing contraception are the ones who are most likely to begin and continue using it. What I am stressing is that all kinds of activity of a legitimating character are required. Some persons are removing IUD's because they have side effects and give discomfort. But many persons are taking them out for quite different reasons. They genuinely wanted the IUD when they received it. They thought that was the balance, but since they have had some doubts.

In Taiwan and most other places, they are attempting to supplement the intra-uterine device, which has been the main reliance in most of the programs, with the contraceptive pill. I received a report on an effort being made in one group of villages and it was not having much success. They could not get women interested. I do not know what the program is in this particular case, but I can say, on the basis of knowing the persons involved, that they probably made a reasonable and intelligent effort to present the pill.

I emphasize Taiwan not only because I know it well, but because the success of a program is more probable there than in other places. Mortality is low. The country is high in the rank of developing countries. There is presently considerable use of contraception. They have an excellent communication network. Everything seems favorable.

Returning to the optimistic side, I think that it is likely, in the next decade, that countries with high birth rates will solve some of these problems, either through the program or by working alone. I have tried to communicate briefly here what has been bothering me this year. I am leaving soon for a tour of various countries, and Asia in particular. I have been reading the reports. This year's reports from those countries in which the programs are having difficulty in beginning are not very good. But they are over the first blush of "isn't this wonderful and we've got this new intra-uterine device," and so forth.

SAMORA: My role in population is recent. In August of this year, I started working with the Ford Foundation in Mexico and Central America. On the basis of this very limited experience, I would like to wear my pessimistic hat. As Mr. Saunders has taught me, an effective program in family planning tends to include effective organization, good record keeping, an excellent information service, a medical follow-up, an available supplier of contraceptives, and an evaluation program. Such a program demonstrates that family planning is very complex. It is not a matter of having IUD's in your pocket and giving them to women. From that point of view, I am somewhat pessimistic in terms of the world situation. In discussing a family program, it is one thing to say that a country has a national program and another thing to find the number of clinics they have and the number and kinds of persons they reach. Mr. Saunders is very aware of this.

In Mexico, there are some excellent clinics under Dr. Edris Rice-Wray. She has been working seven or eight years and serves 11,000 women. About 14 other clinics are to be built within the next year. Considering that Mexico has 45 million persons and Edris Rice-Wray has reached 11,000 women in seven years, this gives me more room for pessimism.

I would like to ask Mr. Saunders two questions. I would like to know if he knows what the potential number of women of childbearing age in the world is and how many of these women are being reached by any contraceptive devices. Secondly, I would like to know what he thinks is the status of the training programs throughout the world. Assuming that trained personnel, such as M.D.'s, are necessary for the successful use of contraceptives and assuming, as Mr. Freedman does, that massive support and legitimation, etc., are necessary, let us suppose that ten countries in the world wanted to begin national programs. What is the status of the personnel? Will there be enough trained doctors to carry out these programs? Certainly, we do not have enough doctors in the United States; I rather doubt that we do in other parts of the world.

SAUNDERS: The demographers use a kind of rule of thumb for estimating the number of women of childbearing ages in the population. It is about a sixth of the population. Therefore, for the world, I would estimate the number of "vulnerable" women would be around 500 to 600 million. How many of these are using modern contraceptive devices? The estimates I gave you on the pills indicate something. Assume they are 100 per cent wrong. They could not be 100 per cent wrong as an overestimate, since that would mean nobody is using the pill. However, if we assume that they are a 100 per cent underestimate, it would still be only 20 million women, which is a tiny fraction. The IUD users certainly are not more than that and probably much less. I would not want to make an estimate, but I would certainly think it is not around 20 million.

So, a relatively small proportion uses IUD's. But I would like to refer to the other point I made. Many couples are not practicing family planning very successfully in countries that have birth rates of 25 or less. The fact that the birth rates are 25 or less indicates that a fairly substantial number of the couples are keeping their fertility down in some way. The alternatives are either they do not have a normal proportion of women who are married and of childbearing ages, they are marrying very late, or they are infertile to a very considerable extent.

Let us take the population of Europe, the United States, Canada, Uruguay, Argentina, and Japan. The total is about a billion persons. I do not think the conditions of abnormal distribution of age groups, or widespread infertility, or late age at marriage would apply broadly over that whole population. So, here is a group of persons that somehow are limiting fertility. In the long run, I do not think they are limiting fertility enough to handle the population growth situation. They still have growth rates of about 1 per cent a year, which demonstrates a doubling time of about 70 years. With a population base in the world of about 3.3 billion, any small percentage of increase is going to result in a lot of persons.

If the rate of increase of the world population could be reduced to the rate of the countries which have birth rates of 25 or less, we would still have a substantial increase of about 30 to 35 million persons every year. The longer we postpone this

249

result, the higher that figure is going to be.

Concerning the pessimism and optimism dilemma, I am very pessimistic. I do not think we are going to do it. On the optimistic side, one might point out that we only recently received the kind of effort, organization, tools, and techniques that are now available.

The program in Taiwan, about which Mr. Freedman is talking, has only been in operation for three or four years. To expect it to have miraculous effects in a short time would be unrealistic. The fact that before we had these techniques populations could control themselves, not through designed programs but through the individual actions of many persons, indicates that there is at least a theoretical possibility that we can have a world with no fertility. All of the things that we are doing, I think, have some small contribution. The effect would be much larger than it has been if the programs and the kinds of legitimating activities of which Mr. Freedman spoke are continued, intensified, and elaborated.

The fact that a government has a program is a legitimating influence. The fact that services are offered in the community indicates an opportunity to talk about them and get ideas into informal channels where they can be accepted and perhaps legitimized by peers, neighbors, friends, and relatives. It is surprising how many persons who have used the clinics in Taiwan and Korea have said that they learned about the program from relatives, friends, and neighbors.

Mr. Samora also asked about the training facilities. I do not think there is yet a clear idea about the types of training we need, the best place to give it, or who should have it. We are still experimenting because this is a new field. It has not had time to shake down. At least there are training programs in the administration of family planning, at the University of Michigan where Mr. Freedman teaches, at Johns Hopkins, University of Chicago, and one or two other institutions. North Carolina and, to some extent, Berkeley have training programs which are very vigorous. Programs are also offered in Chile. The medical profession is changing rapidly by incorporating more information about sex, reproduction, and family planning into medical training and by offering refresher courses. There is some rudimentary training in programs we have tried to start in Egypt at the Universities of Cairo and Alexandria. Although attention is being given and a number of training opportunities are being expanded, it is my judgment that we are not clear about the procedures and we really do not know what kinds of training are best. The present situation, frankly, is experimental.

CONFERENCE PARTICIPANTS

BARRETT, DONALD N., Associate Professor of Sociology, Director, Institute for the Study of Latin American Population, University of Notre Dame

CARNEY, THOMAS P., Senior Vice President, G. D. Searle Co., Chicago

CHRISTENSEN, HAROLD T., Professor of Sociology, Purdue University

CROSSON, FREDERICK J., Professor of General Program, Associate Director, Philosophic Institute for the Study of Artificial Intelligence, University of Notre Dame

D'ANTONIO, WILLIAM V., Head and Professor, Department of Sociology, University of Notre Dame

DUFFY, BENEDICT J., Professor, Department of Preventive Medicine, Tufts University Medical School, Boston

DUNNE, JOHN, C.S.C., Professor, Department of Theology, University of Notre Dame

FREEDMAN, RONALD, Professor of Sociology, Director, The Population Studies Center, University of Michigan

GREELEY, ANDREW M., Senior Study Director, National Opinion Research Center, Chicago

HAGMAIER, GEORGE, C.S.P., Chaplain, Harvard-Radcliff Newman Center, Cambridge, Massachusetts

HILL, REUBEN, Professor of Sociology, Director, Minnesota Family Study Center, University of Minnesota

IMBIORSKI, WALTER, The Cana Conference, Chicago

JOHNSON, VIRGINIA, Washington University Medical School, St. Louis

KANE, JOHN J., Professor of Sociology, University of Notre Dame

KOSA, JOHN, Associate Director, Family Health Care Program, Harvard Medical School

KUTZ, STANLEY, C.S.B., Professor of Theology, St. Michael's College, University of Toronto

LIU, WILLIAM T., Professor of Sociology, Director, Institute for the Study of Population and Social Change, University of Notre Dame

MASTERS, WILLIAM, Washington University Medical School, St. Louis

MCCORMICK, RICHARD, S.J., Bellarmine School of Theology of Loyola University, North Aurora, Illinois

MCDONOUGH, THOMAS B., Calvert House, University of Chicago

MCHUGH, JAMES T., Director, Family Life Bureau, United States Catholic Conference, Inc., Washington, D.C.

PERKIN, GORDON, Medical Advisor, Population Program, Ford Foundation

POTVIN, RAYMOND, Associate Professor of Sociology, Catholic University of America

ROBERTSON, LEON S., Research Associate, Family Health Care Program, Harvard Medical School

RYDER, NORMAN B., Professor of Sociology, Director, Population Research, University of Wisconsin

SAMORA, JULIAN, Professor of Sociology, University of Notre Dame

SAUNDERS, LYLE, Associate Program Director, Population Program, Ford Foundation

SCHLITZER, ALBERT L., C.S.C., Head and Professor, Department of Theology, University of Notre Dame

SHUSTER, GEORGE N., Assistant to the President, Director, Center for the Study of Man in Contemporary Society, University of Notre Dame

SOUTHAM, ANNA L., Medical Advisor, Population Program, Ford Foundation

STRODTBECK, FRED L., Associate Professor of Sociology and Psychology, Director, Social Psychology Laboratory, University of Chicago

STUART, MARTHA, Martha Stuart Communication Inc., Consultant, Planned Parenthood and World Population, New York

SUSSMAN, MARVIN B., Head and Professor of Sociology, Western Reserve University

TAMNEY, JOSEPH B., Head, Department of Sociology, Marquette University

THOMAS, JOHN L., S.J., Resident Scholar, Cambridge Center for Social Studies, Cambridge, Massachusetts

VALENTE, MICHAEL F., Department of Religion, Columbia University

WESTOFF, CHARLES F., Head, Department of Sociology, Associate Director, Office of Population Research, Princeton University